SO YOU WANT TO BE A DOCTOR?

A GUIDE FOR
PROSPECTIVE AND
CURRENT MEDICAL
STUDENTS IN AUSTRALIA

SO YOU WANT TO BE A DOCTOR?

A GUIDE FOR PROSPECTIVE AND CURRENT MEDICAL STUDENTS IN AUSTRALIA

KERRY BREEN

AUSTRALIAN SCHOLARLY

Revised 2020 edition by
Australian Scholarly Publishing Pty Ltd
7 Lt Lothian St Nth, North Melbourne, Vic 3051
Tel: 03 9329 6963 / Fax: 03 9329 5452
enquiry@scholarly.info / www.scholarly.info

First published 2011 by
the Australian Council on Educational Research

ISBN 978-1-925984-76-7

Cover design: Wayne Saunders

CONTENTS

FOREWORD

Contemplating medical studies can be daunting, exciting and above all confusing. Advice from family, friends, current medical students and medical graduates is often helpful but can also be conflicting. The growth in new medical schools in the last decade each with subtly different expectations can also add to the disorientation that the prospective medical student may feel. In this clear, comprehensive and fully revised guide Dr Kerry Breen provides definitive answers to all of your questions and makes a complex process clearer. This book gives aspiring medical students the confidence they need to approach their preparation for medical school entry. Dr Breen covers graduate versus undergraduate courses, course length, aptitude tests and interview processes with cogent and succinct overviews. For those successful graduates, this book also provides important tips about the internship year and subsequent career planning. This book is a must for students and families who need help to navigate the increasing complexity of medical school entry.

Professor Michelle Leech MBBS (Hons), FRACP, PhD
Deputy Dean and Head of Medical Course
Faculty of Medicine Nursing and Health Sciences
Monash University

PREFACE

A revised edition of this book is needed for several reasons. Since the first edition was published, new medical schools have been established in Australia and some of the existing ones have altered their curricula. In addition several have altered their student selection methods in the light of further research. Local and international studies continue to focus on the well-being of medical students and recent medical graduates and on the factors that can prevent student and junior doctor distress and ill-health so the revision provides an opportunity to update the book on these matters. In addition, in this electronic age, the websites of institutions and organisations are fluid and web links can disappear overnight much to the reader's frustration. All the websites referenced have been checked and where necessary updated.

Students face a number of hurdles as well as difficult decisions in seeking to enrol in a medical school. The hurdles include national entry or aptitude tests (UCAT or GAMSAT) and probing interviews. They must consider the financial debt that most modern university students gradually accumulate. They have also greater choices, given the recent growth in number and variety of medical schools in Australia, but this does not simplify their decisions. Students must decide whether to seek entry into medicine as a school leaver or to pursue another university degree first, whether to apply to a medical school in another state, and whether to accept financial support via a medical school place that is 'bonded', i.e. will tie them to a mandated period, possibly years, of work in a designated area after all training is completed.

A small but consistent proportion of students later regret their decision to become doctors. Much has been written about the stresses of medical student life, the burden of medical practice, and some of the health consequences for students and doctors. Those consequences were previously addressed primarily in the context of the pressure of study or the job, rather than the vulnerability of the individual student or doctor. This emphasis has shifted as research indicates that personal factors in the student or doctor, including childhood experiences, temperament and personality may contribute to stress and distress. These studies also indicate that distressed or unwell students and doctors avoid seeking help for a variety of reasons, not the least being fear of stigmatisation, and yet most can be helped by early intervention and will go on to enjoy rewarding careers. At the same time, there has been renewed attention to support for stressed junior doctors and on improving their work environment. Since the first edition, there has been an increased focus on the resilience of medical students and doctors and whether resilience is innate or can be taught or enhanced.

Ten years ago in a review of the value of assessment, via interview, of non-cognitive traits (i.e. qualities other than intellectual or academic capacity including elements such as innate communication skills, self-awareness, empathy, and capacity for independent learning) in selecting medical students, the authors argued that the interview and selection process 'should assist prospective applicants to make informed decisions based on a reflective self-appraisal' thus 'encouraging an informed decision to apply to medical school'.* I felt then that their advice about 'an informed decision' was very important and adopted it as the key theme of the first edition, an approach maintained in this edition. As is explained, coming to such an informed decision is also a means of better understanding your reasons for choosing medicine and of preparing yourself for the selection processes ahead.

If I am correct in this emphasis on making *an informed decision*, many good things may follow. If your application is successful, you will enter medical school reasonably well informed as to what lies ahead and you

---

* Benbassat, J, Baumal, R. 'Uncertainties in the selection of applicants for medical school.' *Advances in Health Sciences Education,* 2007: 12: 509–21.

can use your medical student days to help create a firm basis for seeking an appropriate work/life balance throughout your career. Some of you who read this book will opt for other careers, careers best suited to your temperament and aspirations, and if so, I hope those careers are satisfying and rewarding. For those medical students who do experience distress in the course of their studies (and some of you surely will), hopefully the information in this book will guide you to early assistance and you will still be able to fulfil your ambition.

Of course the book does more than address the stresses and difficulties that some students experience. It outlines why most doctors in Australia find their careers to be emotionally and intellectually rewarding. It also covers the relevant information a prospective medical student will need in regard to Australia's medical schools, their selection processes and how best to prepare for these. In addition, as medical students have expressed a desire to have early access to information about career choices after graduation, the book addresses this topic.

While still a single author book, I have again been able to obtain generous input from current medical students and recent medical graduates as well as more senior doctors whose careers have given them great experience in teaching, mentoring and counselling students and junior doctors.

Kerry J Breen
2020

ACKNOWLEDGEMENTS

During the writing of both editions, I recalled my own experiences of medical school and postgraduate training, especially the very positive influences of some outstanding teachers and role models. Although I chose eventually to be a physician and not a surgeon, the most warmly recalled role models from my student days were a cardiothoracic surgeon, a neurosurgeon and two paediatric surgeons, as well as two excellent registrars. In a small way the book is a tribute to all those people. Thus I first acknowledge these and many other role models, mentors and colleagues from whom I have learned so much over many years.

In addition to my own experiences, the final product owes an enormous debt to a large group of people in Australia and around the world who have researched and published in the fields of medical student selection, education, health and well-being, and in the field of junior doctor well-being. Their work is referred to throughout the book.

The scope of the book has been widened and its content enhanced by the generous input of an editorial advisory panel, all of whose members read and commented on two drafts of the manuscript. They guided me to additional sources of information, identified my errors and biases and made very helpful suggestions to improve the text. The membership of that panel together with a little background information about each is given below. I am very grateful for their assistance.

Ms Theanne Walters and Dr Barbara Demediuk read the revised manuscript and I am grateful for their helpful comments.

Finally I am indebted to Nick Walker and the team at Australian Scholarly Publishing for their excellent work; once again it was a great pleasure to work with them.

EDITORIAL ADVISORY PANEL

Professor Jochanan Benbassat, internal medicine specialist and past Chair of Medical Education at the Hebrew University Hadassah Medical School in Israel.

Dr Claude Dennis, a graduate from the University of Sydney and currently an intern at St George's Hospital, Kogarah, NSW.

Dr Kym Jenkins, immediate past president of Royal Australian and New Zealand College Psychiatrists and past medical director of the Victorian Doctors Health Program.

Dr Jacinta Mogg, tutor at Monash University Medical School and past Clinical Subdean at St Vincent's Hospital Clinical School of the University of Melbourne.

Dr Ruth Sladek, senior lecturer in Medical Education, Flinders University's College of Medicine and Public Health. She held the role of Chair of the Medical Course Admissions Committee at Flinders for over 7 years.

Associate Professor Ashley Watson, infectious diseases expert and medical educator at the Australian National University Medical School and Canberra Hospital.

Ms Ellie Watson, third year medical student at Deakin University Medical School at Geelong, Victoria.

ABOUT THE AUTHOR

When he enrolled to study medicine at the University of Melbourne, Kerry Breen's background was a little unusual. Born and raised in a remote Victorian rural community, his primary schooling was partly by correspondence and partly at very small one teacher schools, where his father was the teacher. His secondary education was mostly undertaken as a boarder at Assumption College in Kilmore, Victoria. After graduating as a doctor via the University of Melbourne, his postgraduate medical training years were spent at St Vincent's Hospital in Melbourne, Royal Prince Alfred Hospital in Sydney and Vanderbilt University Hospital in the USA. He worked as a general physician and gastroenterologist at St Vincent's Hospital, Melbourne for most of his clinical career. During these years he was deeply involved in teaching medical students and in supervising and supporting doctors in training.

Via his appointment to the Medical Practitioners Board of Victoria (now superseded by the Medical Board of Australia), on which he served for 19 years, he developed interests in the ethical issues of everyday medical practice and in the health and well-being of medical students and doctors. He has served as President of the Medical Practitioners Board of Victoria, President of the Australian Medical Council, Chairman of the Australian Health Ethics Committee of the National Health and Medical Research Council, Chairman of the Board of the Victorian Doctors Health Program and member of the Australian Research Integrity Committee. He is a co-author of the book *Good Medical Practice; Professionalism, Ethics and Law*, the fourth edition of which was published by the Australian Medical Council in 2016 and is the author of two medical biographies and a memoir. He currently holds an appointment as Adjunct Professor in the Department of Forensic Medicine at Monash University.

LIST OF ABBREVIATIONS

ACER	Australian Council for Educational Research
ADF	Australian Defence Force
AHPRA	Australian Health Practitioners Regulation Agency
AMA	Australian Medical Association
AMC	Australian Medical Council
AMSA	Australian Medical Students' Association
ATAR	Australian Tertiary Admission Rank
ATO	Australian Taxation Office
BMedSc	Bachelor of Medical Science
BMSt	Bachelor of Medical Studies
BMP	Bonded Medical Places
CMO	career medical officer
CPMEC	Confederation of Postgraduate Medical Education Councils
CSP	Commonwealth supported places
DHAS	Doctors' Health Advisory Services
GAMSAT	Graduate Australian Medical School Admissions Test
GE	graduate entry (medical course)
GEMSAS	Graduate Entry Medical School Admission System
GP	general practitioner
GPA	grade point average
HECS	Higher Education Contribution Scheme
HIV	human immunodeficiency virus
IELTS	International English Language Testing System
IES	Indigenous Entry Stream

IMS	international medical student
ISAT	International Student Admissions Test
JMP	Joint Medical Program
MABEL	Medicine in Australia: Balancing Employment and Life
MBA	Medical Board of Australia
MBBS	Bachelor of Medicine and Bachelor of Surgery
MCAT	Medical College Admission Test (North America)
MD	Doctor of Medicine (postgraduate medical degree)
MMI	multi-station mini-interview
OSCE	objective structured clinical examination
PBL	problem-based learning
PGY	Postgraduate Year
PhD	Doctor of Philosophy
PQA	personal qualities assessment
RACP	Royal Australasian College of Physicians
RACS	Royal Australasian College of Surgeons
UG	undergraduate entry (medical course)
UCAT	University Clinical Aptitude Test
VMO	visiting medical officer

INTRODUCTION

Although it is now commonly stated that people should expect to have more than one career in a lifetime, this is probably not so for most doctors. Thus if you are thinking about studying to become a doctor, you need to be aware that you are probably deciding on the future direction of your entire working life – in other words you are about to make a very important decision. However, you should also take note that medical graduates have a wide range of career paths, some only tangentially related to health care. In addition, it is not unknown for doctors to completely change career direction. Some later train to practise law or become authors, journalists or playwrights while others go in to politics, business, the media or the religious ministry.

The key aim of this short book is to help you think through your initial decision. The book does not try to make your decision for you; instead it gives you some things to ask yourself about your career choice and provides information that might help answer some of the questions that commonly arise. These questions create the structure of the book as is shown in the list of contents, commencing with 'What makes a good doctor and what is expected of doctors?'

The book is divided into five sections. The first section addresses the issue of how a young person considering a career in medicine can become confident that she or he is likely to enjoy the work of being a doctor and become a competent and good doctor. The next section provides information about the existing Australian medical schools. It describes the processes used by the medical schools to select applicants for entry and outlines suggestions for preparation for these processes. As the processes for entry and the nature of the courses available vary across Australia (e.g. in duration, school-leaver entry versus university graduate entry, and rural emphasis), this section also covers these aspects and provides sources of more detailed information. The third section provides information about the structure and content of the medical course while the fourth section describes the typical life of the medical student of today so that potential students can get some idea of what lies ahead, especially in terms of workloads, stresses and financial burdens. Here the reader will also find tips for success once accepted into a medical course and directions as to where help is available if student life proves difficult. The final section outlines what the intern year involves and opens up the topic of career paths for medical graduates after completion of the intern* year. In each section, additional issues that may be relevant only to certain subgroups of people considering a career in medicine (e.g. Indigenous students, students with children, students with disabilities, international students) are also addressed.

Entry into medicine and into some other university courses is highly competitive. That competition is not always fair to all Australian high school students as data show that success can be related to choice and location of high school (private vs public, urban vs rural) and to parental economic and educational status. An additional aim of this book is to strive to produce a more level playing field in so far as seeking to have all applicants to medical school equally informed about selection processes, sources of support and other matters.

Surveys in Australia and overseas have identified a significant minority of medical students and doctors who experience distress and health problems in response to the challenges of student life and later of clinical practice. In acknowledgement of these findings and as a means of seeking preventive approaches as early in the career of prospective doctors as possible, I have explored these issues in some depth. Sections 4 and 5 examine what is known about why some students and some doctors appear

---

* The term 'intern' or 'internship' in the medical context refers to a compulsory year of predominantly hospital based practical experience, obtained under supervision, that all medical graduates must complete before they can be granted general registration by the Medical Board of Australia.

to be more vulnerable to stress, describe the experiences that are most likely to be stressful, discuss the importance of self-care, and provide guidance about when and where to seek help.

Apart from the information provided in this book, there are other sources to consider. A particularly good source of information, updated regularly, is the website of the Australian Medical Students' Association (www.amsa.org.au), where you will find a number of guides on topics including applying for medicine, starting the medical course and the intern year. There is also advice about maintaining one's health and about pitfalls in the use of social media. The Australian Medical Association provides advice in a document headed 'Becoming a doctor'.[1] You might also wish to seek advice from career advisers and counsellors in your school and/or your university. You should also seek out and attend university open days. Some medical schools conduct regular information sessions for prospective students and information about these sessions can be found on the medical school websites (see Section 2).

MAKING AN INFORMED DECISION

The key aim of my book and especially this section is to help you to decide whether you are likely to enjoy the work of being a doctor and whether you feel you have the attributes to become a good doctor. You will find that there are no absolute ways of being sure about your decision but at least when you make it, you should be well informed not only about the rewarding and enjoyable things involved in a career in medicine but also some of the potentially negative aspects.

1.1 What makes a good doctor and what is expected of doctors?

Much has been written in recent years about the qualities required of a 'good doctor'. Over the same time, medical school selection methods have been altered in anticipation that the selection process will result in a higher proportion of graduates who become 'good doctors' and a smaller proportion of problem doctors. That there are many factors, in addition to the selection process, that will help produce good doctors seem at times to be overlooked. As discussed later, these factors include the contributions, via education, mentoring and role-modelling at medical school and in subsequent postgraduate training as well as the effects of experience and maturation on your development as a doctor. As a prospective medical student you should not be intimidated by the detail contained in these descriptions of the good doctor.

While the majority of medical graduates work in clinical practice, there is a broad range of ways in which medical graduates can be employed. When commentators write about the desirable qualities of a 'good doctor' they have in mind those doctors (the vast majority) who have to be competent in clinical practice and feel rewarded with spending most of their time working directly with people who are unwell. These desirable qualities will be less central to a successful career in medical fields where direct patient contact generally does not occur or occurs infrequently (e.g. pathology and its various branches, medical administration, laboratory medicine and medical research). As McManus and colleagues wrote:

> The immediate job characteristics of a neurosurgeon, a public health physician, a histopathologist and a psychiatrist vary almost as much as being a doctor itself differs from being an airline pilot, an accountant or a museum curator.[1]

Despite this wider range of eventual career options it must also be emphasised that in the Australian health care system and its medical training scheme, all medical graduates have to complete an intern year and usually some additional clinical years working closely with patients in public hospitals and some private hospitals before moving into any field that has little or no direct patient contact. Thus all medical graduates need to have or acquire a high level of communication skills no matter what field of medicine is their eventual destination.

Later in the book, factors in your make up that might influence your choice of career in medicine after graduation will be considered. For the moment, as most prospective medical students seem initially drawn towards the caring role of the medical practitioner, it is helpful to describe here the ideal qualities sought in modern doctors. These qualities have been primarily developed and described by doctors and by others, especially by those who are drawn to the study of ethics in medicine. In Australia, the national health consumer organisation, the Consumer Health Forum, has also given its input into what are considered to be desirable qualities in doctors. From combining these various views, prospective medical students can be told that the Australian community hopes that its doctors will demonstrate in their *professional* lives the following qualities: respectfulness, a capacity for self-reflection, honesty and truthfulness, fidelity and trustworthiness, integrity, compassion, empathy, collegiality and capability for teamwork, discernment, judgement and appreciation of the importance of privacy and confidentiality.[2] Doctors also need to be conscientious and thorough, be good communicators, have excellent interpersonal skills, be capable of making decisions, and have the mental resilience and emotional stability to perform well in stressful situations.[3] Australian medical students agree with and accept these expectations, rating empathy, motivation to be a good doctor, having good communication skills, being ethically sound and being honest as the most important qualities.[4] These qualities are in addition to the required knowledge, practical skills and clinical competence that practising doctors need.

Doctors registered to practise in Australia are obliged to abide by a code of conduct issued by the Medical Board of Australia, it is entitled *Good Medical Practice: A Code of Conduct for Doctors in Australia.*[5] A short document, it provides a very useful picture of what is expected of doctors in clinical practice. Under the heading, *Professional Values and Qualities of Doctors*, the Code describes what the medical profession *and* the Australian community expect of their doctors as follows:

> While individual doctors have their own personal beliefs and values, there are certain professional values on which all doctors are expected to base their practice. Doctors have a duty to make the care of patients their first concern and to practise medicine safely and effectively. They must be ethical and trustworthy. Patients trust their doctors because they believe that, in addition to being competent, their

doctor will not take advantage of them and will display qualities such as integrity, truthfulness, dependability and compassion. Patients also rely on their doctors to protect their confidentiality. Doctors have a responsibility to protect and promote the health of individuals and the community.

Good medical practice is patient-centred. It involves doctors understanding that each patient is unique, and working in partnership with their patients, adapting what they do to address the needs and reasonable expectations of each patient. This includes cultural awareness: being aware of their own culture and beliefs and respectful of the beliefs and cultures of others, recognising that these cultural differences may impact on the doctor–patient relationship and on the delivery of health services. Good communication underpins every aspect of good medical practice.

Professionalism embodies all the qualities described here, and includes self-awareness and self-reflection. Doctors are expected to reflect regularly on whether they are practising effectively, on what is happening in their relationships with patients and colleagues, and on their own health and wellbeing. They have a duty to keep their skills and knowledge up to date, refine and develop their clinical judgement as they gain experience, and contribute to their profession.

Our society also places additional expectations in regard to the *private* lives of doctors. This is exemplified by the 'good character' provisions of medical registration (e.g. a doctor can be refused registration or be de-registered if he or she is convicted and jailed for a serious crime unrelated to medical practice). Other manifestations of society's expectations of doctors that go beyond the confines of medical practice can be seen in the considerable trust placed in doctors; e.g. to witness signatures for passports and other important documents. In addition, doctors and medical students are expected to adhere to professional standards in their use of social media.[6]

1.2 But how can I be sure that I will be able to meet these expectations? How do I assess myself as to whether I am really suited to being a doctor?

There are no certain answers to these questions other than to point out some personal features that might suggest you could be unsuited to a career in medicine as discussed below. There are a range of aptitude tests and tools for assessing temperament and personality that may be suggested to students and that you may be tempted to seek out. It is difficult to envisage any harm, other than financial, arising in taking such tests but you should avoid making too much of the results in choosing your career, as their usefulness in predicting success has not been demonstrated. They might be better looked upon as tools that can help you understand the sort of person you are.

To enjoy a lifetime in clinical medicine you will need an attitude of being interested in other people, a capacity to place the needs of others ahead of your own, and a willingness to work hard when required. If you are serious about becoming a doctor and if you are going to be well-prepared for the interviews that the medical school selection involves, you need to undertake some honest self-reflection. What do you think are your strengths and weaknesses? Could any of your strengths create challenges for you? For example, if you see yourself as very conscientious and capable of empathising with patients, could this put you at risk of burnout? Hopefully such reflection will be a little easier after you have read this book.

If you are selected, you should be confident that you can meet what may seem to be quite daunting expected attributes. In the four to six years of medical education and the additional six to eight years of postgraduate training, there is ample opportunity to develop and/or enhance the qualities that are desired of doctors in clinical practice. Most young people change as they mature and are positively influenced by life's experiences, education and training, and good role modelling and mentorship. A larger problem sometimes flows from young people being too conscientious and immersing themselves too heavily in the work of the profession, thereby putting themselves at risk of troubled lives and troubled relationships. Thus you will also need to learn to become aware of your own needs and not ignore them.

You might be unsuited to studying medicine if you have already found the study expected in secondary school or your undergraduate university course to be very stressful. This is especially so if you have used alcohol and/or drugs as a release from those stresses and tension. You might be unsuited if you feel that the choice of a career in medicine is being thrust upon you by family or community expectations rather than this being your own first choice. If your reasons for considering medicine are based predominantly on the notions of the career being glamorous and bringing high social status and high income then you should think again and do some more research into what most doctors really do and really earn, how many hours a day are worked (including, for some, being on continuous call), and how many demands are involved to earn certain levels of income.

Studies of the experience of stress in medical students and in new medical graduates have identified some factors within the individual student or doctor that may make that person more liable than their peers to become distressed, anxious or depressed. This material is covered in more detail later in the book. The traits that have been identified include introversion (shyness), non-joining behaviour (loner) and neuroticism (see footnote page 18). The authors of these studies have not suggested that people with such traits should not study medicine; indeed a mild degree of any of such traits might make the person a very conscientious doctor. The point of mentioning these studies here is to help you reflect on your own personality and temperament so you are as well informed as possible before taking on an exacting tertiary course and a demanding professional life. Knowing and understanding more about yourself is likely to make you a better doctor and help you adopt appropriate coping strategies if you ever do find yourself being unduly stressed.

The assessment methods used for selecting medical students (see Section 2) are designed not only to ensure that you have the academic capacity to cope with a demanding curriculum but also to seek to determine that you are suited to a career as a doctor. The latter include searching interviews and evaluation of your 'non-academic' or 'non-cognitive'* traits. Enrolling in medical school is a serious decision both for you and for the university. Your own decision needs to be a well-informed one.[7] A central intention of this book is to assist you in this. The process of informing your decision will not only help you to make the best decision but should also stimulate you to think through why you want to become a doctor. By engaging in such thinking, you are at the same time preparing yourself for the interviews you will face during the selection process.

1.3 Do I know what doctors really do? How can I find out?

Most people gain their impressions of the work of doctors from (a) family, friends or acquaintances (b) personal interaction with the health care system and (c) the media, especially via popular television shows. You may also have had an opportunity to hear a doctor answer questions at a careers session at your school. None of these sources can be complete or fully reliable, with the media in particular tending to glamorise clinical practice. Accounts about the work of doctors provided via social media may also be unreliable and unrepresentative of the lives of most doctors.

_____

* 'Non-cognitive' or 'non-academic' traits include qualities such as innate communication skills, empathy, capacity for independent learning, decision making, self-awareness, ability to work in teams, and integrity. ('Non-cognitive' in this context is a simple shorthand term used to distinguish such qualities from cognitive or academic capacity and achievement.) One dictionary defines empathy as an 'appreciative perception or understanding'. Medical writers have described empathy variously as 'the ability to understand the perspectives and emotions of others and to communicate that you understand these perspectives and emotions' or 'a capacity and motivation to take in patient/colleague perspective and sense associated feelings – the ability to generate a safe/understanding atmosphere'. Research indicates that women students and doctors are naturally more empathic than men (*Academic Medicine,* 2017 Oct., 92(10): 1464–71 and *Academic Medicine,* 2015 Jan., 90(1): 105–11). It is unclear whether empathy can be fostered through education and mentoring. Some studies report reduction in empathy in doctors who are stressed and burnt out.

Open days at universities can also be useful. In addition your local or family doctor or another doctor or specialist known to your family will very likely be happy to make time to talk with you. A teacher at your school may also be able to assist in arranging for this to happen. If offered, do not hesitate to talk to such a doctor as there is a very strong tradition and expectation in the medical profession of helping to train future doctors. Most schools promote the practice of a short time in 'work experience' and it may be possible to arrange time at your nearest hospital, general practice or specialist clinic.

A number of doctors have written personal accounts of their professional experiences and some clinical psychologists who have worked closely with young doctors have also written enlightening accounts of what they learnt about the lives of those doctors. The books listed below include examples of both categories of book and are well worth reading for their insights. Reading even one or two of them may encourage you to think more deeply as to why you are seeking a life as a doctor, and if so, will help you prepare for the interviews that all Australian medical schools now conduct with prospective students.

What It Takes to Be a Doctor: An Insider's Guide. Ranjana Srivastava. Simon & Schuster, Australia, 2018. Dr Ranjana Srivastava is a Melbourne-based oncologist and writer. She has written a personal account of her own career together with an insightful description of the highs and lows of becoming a doctor. Of its many strengths, the one that may be of greatest help to potential medical students is the wise advice she has for those who feel pushed into medicine through parental pressure.

Also Human: The Inner Lives of Doctors. Caroline Elton. Penguin Random House, UK, 2018. Caroline Elton is an occupational psychologist with extensive experience in helping distressed doctors in the UK and in providing careers guidance. There are sufficient similarities between the UK medical education and hospital systems and those in Australia for her insights to be directly relevant in Australia. While her book focuses primarily on the cases of individual doctors in difficulty, mostly junior doctors still in training, it provides deep insight into the predictable and unpredictable stresses that all young doctors may face.

Becoming a Doctor: From Student to Specialist, Doctor-Writers Share Their Experiences. Lee Gutkind (ed.). WW Norton & Co, New York, NY, 2010. This contains personal accounts from around twenty doctors who describe various facets of their transition from medical student to practice in their chosen field. All of the doctors have had 'side' careers as serious writers and this enhances the beauty and clarity of their writing – and of course makes them not quite your 'average' doctor. The accounts, although drawn only from experience in USA, can be reasonably translated to similar experiences of Australian medical students and doctors. A particularly valuable aspect of this book is that many of the writers describe not only the 'highs' of their experience but also the 'lows'. Because of this balance, I recommend it to all prospective medical students.

The Pen and the Stethoscope. Leah Kaminsky (ed.). Scribe Publications, Melbourne, 2010. This contains real life and fictional short stories written by doctors from around the world, five of whom are Australian medical graduates, including the editor. The real life accounts include several stories built around situations faced shortly after graduation where the doctor-authors honestly explore their own feelings and emotions, and at the same time demonstrate empathy with the dilemmas faced by the patients. Many of the stories have been published before and the writing is outstanding.

How to Survive in Medicine, Personally and Professionally. Jenny Firth-Cozens with Jamie Harrison. Wiley-Blackwell, Oxford, 2010. Dr Firth-Cozens is a UK based academic clinical psychologist who has studied the experiences of large numbers of medical students and young doctors through their careers and with a colleague has written a very informative and wise book about the pressures students and doctors will face in their professional and private lives, and how to prevent or cope with problems.

1.4 What hours do doctors work, how hard do they work and what do they earn?

The hours worked by doctors vary considerably depending upon the type of medical practice, whether the doctor chooses to work part time or full time, and whether there are on call and after-hours responsibilities. The most recently available Australian data show that the average hours worked per week were highest for registrars (advanced trainees) at 46 h, followed by hospital medical officers (also trainees and including interns) at 45 h, specialists at 42 h and general practitioners at 37 h. These figures also showed that there had been a 12% drop in hours worked in all groups over the last nine years. However, these are averages only and include those doctors who opt to work part-time. A significant proportion of doctors work over 50 hours per week, especially trainees, a workload that is now deemed unsafe.[8]

Many specialist doctors in private practice remain on call for their practice continuously other than when annual leave is taken. If the specialty has a large component involving care of patients admitted to hospital (e.g. all fields of surgery, obstetrics, much of internal medicine and some areas of psychiatry) then the doctor is rarely completely free of professional responsibilities. A very similar situation applies to general practitioners working in remote or rural areas where after-hours locum (deputising) services are not available. The demands of medical practice relate not just to hours worked but also to the nature of the clinical responsibilities involved, both in routine working hours and after hours.

For doctors on call, a common situation for trainees and those working independently, the expectations are high. You must be prepared to drop everything in response to a call, you must not be too distant from your workplace and you must be sober so the use of alcohol must be minimal or nil. These responsibilities sometimes come as shock to young doctors while for more experienced doctors, they can be a reason for stress and inappropriate coping mechanisms.

Some qualifications must be placed on data about doctors' earnings. At times the media publicise the total amounts of reimbursement paid by Medicare to doctors in various fields. For some specialities the amounts may seem to be very large but this does not take into account the widely varying overhead costs of different specialties. For general practitioners and other medical specialists, overheads (staff, rent, insurance, supplies etc.) are usually of the order of 50% of gross or pre-tax earnings while in areas of investigative medicine such as radiology and pathology, the cost of equipment and staff makes up a much larger proportion.

A better way of looking at what doctors earn is to examine their incomes expressed as hourly rates of remuneration, after expenses and overheads but before tax. On this basis, the most recently available data for specialists (not including general practitioners) show a wide range of earnings within any specialty and between specialties. At the upper end are orthopaedic surgeons whose average hourly earnings are around $260 per hour followed by urologists and radiologists while at the lower end are rheumatologists, neurologists and endocrinologists at around $160 per hour.[9] It is clear that incomes for those specialists who undertake procedures (i.e. surgical operations and investigational procedures such as endoscopies and cardiac catheterisation) are clustered well above those of non-procedural specialists such as physicians and psychiatrists.* Other factors influencing earnings are gender (women doctors earn less than men) and whether a specialist works in private practice only, in both private and public practice, or in the public system solely. For general practitioners, the average remuneration rate in 2015 (again after expenses and before tax) was $116 per hour. Earlier studies have shown a wide spread of general practitioner incomes, being higher if there was a lack of GPs in an area, if the doctor was self-employed, and if GPs took their own after hours calls.

---

* In Australia, the term physician is generally reserved for those trained in some aspect of internal medicine (cardiology, neurology etc) in contrast with the USA where the term physician is usually applied to all medical graduates. In the USA, the equivalent term for the Australian physician is internist. Psychiatrists are medical graduates who then specialise in the diagnosis and treatment of mental illness.

The gender gap in remuneration has been documented in Australia, UK and USA.[10] While it is partially explained by women doctors' choice of field of practice, their propensity to offer more time to each patient, and hours worked, there remains a structural gap in pay as well as barriers to advancement of women doctors' careers.

The salaries of junior doctors (i.e. doctors in training) are addressed in Section 2.23.

1.5 Should I be concerned about finding work as a doctor?

There has been a marked increase in the number of medical schools and the number of medical graduates in Australia over the last twenty years but to date there has been no evidence that new domestic graduates cannot find work. Government policy remains that all new domestic graduates are guaranteed an intern position, thereby ensuring subsequent full registration with the Medical Board of Australia and the freedom to seek work anywhere in Australia. Presently having a medical degree offers considerable vocational security.

Predicting the Australian medical workforce needs and career opportunities is discussed in more detail in Section 5. Experience suggests that any undersupply of doctors will not be uniformly distributed as historically in Australia, and elsewhere,[11] it has been difficult to attract doctors to work in remote and rural areas and to work in some of the less popular fields of medical practice.

In more popular fields, competition for training positions may make it difficult to obtain your first choice of post graduate training.[12] The possibility that the pressure to obtain a training post and to progress in that training may be contributing to unhealthy working styles (e.g. through working extended and unrostered hours to impress supervisors) and to anxiety and depression in junior doctors has been identified as a matter of concern.[13] This issue is discussed in more detail in later Sections.

1.6 Are there any barriers to women studying medicine?

Women represent more than half the number of medical students enrolling and then graduating in Australia and in many other countries. Thus it is clear that there are no barriers at these two levels. Increasingly women graduates are entering into all fields of medical practice so it is also true to say that there is no field or specialty that is closed to women doctors. However, women remain under-represented in surgery and some other fields. Reasons for this remain unclear but are likely multifactorial. Difficulties or obstacles that women doctors might face during postgraduate training are discussed in Section 5.

1.7 What do doctors say influenced them to study medicine?

Commonly reported motivating factors include wanting to help people, being good at science subjects, having always wanted to be a doctor, wanting an interesting, secure and challenging job,[14] and being influenced by family and friends, especially if one or both parents are doctors.[15] However, as a prospective medical student, you should not be concerned if any of these factors are not foremost in mind. Some of these reports have been compiled from responses made long after entering medical school and may not accurately reflect the state of mind of the person at the point of entering medicine. In addition, some of the claimed motivating factors may have been expressed because of their social acceptability.

It is probably socially unacceptable to admit that attractions to study medicine include social prestige, money and success, even when these factors are indeed at work.[16] Encouragingly, the UK report that observed those factors also observed that over a six-year medical course, a 'vocational outlook emerged' and the desire for money, prestige and success diminished.

A large group of 16–17-year-olds attending a national information conference for prospective medical students in the UK participated in a study of their motivations and interests. The study used a questionnaire specially designed to reduce the possibility of students providing socially desirable answers. Four broad dimensions likely to have influenced career choice were identified, viz. (a) a desire to help others, (b) a need to be indispensable, (c) a wish to be a scientist and (d) being respected by society. The authors added

> To a fairly large extent these factors can be explained in terms of personality, learning styles, and demographic factors, although no doubt there are many other events in the lives of our participants, such as individual experience of illness, which also make them want to become doctors.[17]

Many medical students are drawn into medicine by having a family member or close relative already in medicine and a smaller number say they have been influenced by their own illness that led to contact with hospitals and doctors.[18] Parental expectations and family and social pressures at times propel academically high achieving young people into studying medicine. As these young people mature, they may realise that they have made the wrong choice.

People who enter medical school after studying and working in a related health field (e.g. pharmacy, physiotherapy or nursing) appear to be drawn in by the attraction of closer and more meaningful contact with patients and broader and more stimulating tasks than their first career choice provided.

Subconscious factors including early life experiences may influence people to take on a career where they care for others. Dr George Valliant, an American psychiatrist, explored this possibility by comparing the childhoods of doctors with a socioeconomically matched group of controls in other professions. He found that the doctors, especially those involved in patient care, were more likely than matched controls in other professions to encounter the problems of poor marriages, misuse of alcohol or drugs, and the need of psychotherapy. More importantly, these problems were not necessarily related to the pressures of medical practice, as he found that the doctors who had experienced the least stable childhoods and adolescence appeared most vulnerable to these hazards.[19] Unhappy childhood experiences may make people very caring and compassionate doctors. These doctors can also overburden themselves with the work of caring and be predisposed to 'burn out' and inappropriate coping strategies such as substance abuse, as well as to illness or even unprofessional conduct. This is discussed in more detail in Sections 4 and 5 where coping with the stresses of being a medical student and a doctor are addressed.

No studies have been published about the career choices or career outcomes of people who wanted to study medicine but who missed out via the selection process. Anecdotally, many initially unsuccessful applicants have later gained a medical student place in Australia or abroad and have gone on to enjoy very happy careers. The message from these stories is that if you are determined on pursuing a career as a doctor, do not give up if you are not initially selected.

1.8 What do doctors most enjoy about their work?

The answers to this question vary according to the age of the doctor, the nature of their practice and their state of well-being when asked. For most doctors in clinical practice, the primary answer is the satisfaction they enjoy via their regular contact with people. From the UK, Firth-Cozens and Harrison report that younger doctors particularly enjoy their work because they feel useful and feel that they are helping patients. They also say that they enjoy getting to know patients. Older doctors say that they enjoy the variety that their work gives them ('every patient is different'), the challenges of diagnosis or caring for patients, and the rewards of teaching others. General (family) practitioners value the fact that they provide continuity of care and enjoy helping and observing entire families of two or three generations. Many doctors also obtain satisfaction through teaching and mentoring medical students and younger doctors. For all doctors in clinical practice, satisfaction comes when one feels one has made a difference to somebody's life and well-being, as for example in making an elusive diagnosis, especially when effective treatment is available.[20]

As explored later in more depth, not all doctors report enjoyment from their work. An international survey reported that only 16% of doctors in the UK, 34% in Ireland and 36% in NZ were happy or very happy with their career choice.[21] Much higher levels of job satisfaction (over 80%) have been reported for Australian doctors (see 1.9 below). Attitudes to work can be influenced by concurrent professional or personal stresses and are much more likely to be negative if the doctor is burnt out or depressed. These reported differences between countries might reflect different health care systems, differences in methodology of the studies, or other influences.

Many doctors choose careers that involve a small or large component of medical research and derive additional satisfaction from this involvement. Involvement in research by doctors is critical to the continuing advances needed to improve the medical care for the community. Opportunities for research experience and training are discussed in Sections 2.25 and 5.12.

1.9 I have read that some doctors are unhappy with their choice of career. Is there any information about why this might be so?

It has long been recognised that not all doctors are contented with their career choice. However, in any profession, be it teaching, the law, banking and the like, some members eventually become disenchanted with their careers. The real question, for doctors and prospective medical students, is whether this discontent or disenchantment could have been predicted in any one individual. One UK study reported that 14% of men and 19% of women regretted the decision to become doctors; the main reasons for that regret included fatigue and exhaustion and dislike of the long hours and on-call responsibilities.[22]

Another UK study followed a large group of medical students who enrolled over a three year period (1991–93) to see if there were markers at entry that might predict unhappiness or dissatisfaction with medicine thirteen years later. In the over 1,500 doctors who completed a detailed questionnaire (some already in general practice and some finishing specialist training), about one fifth were unhappy in their jobs. No correlations were found between unhappiness and information recorded at entry to medical school, information that included personal statements as to why applicants sought to study medicine and reports from the applicants' referees. It was concluded that these statements and reports, which were intended to assess motivation, interest and commitment to a medical career, could not identify doctors who would be dissatisfied with their medical career.[23]

Until recently there had been little research into the job satisfaction of Australian doctors. A small proportion of Australian doctors report that they are sorry that they chose to be doctors. Two surveys of the health and well-being of junior doctors in Australia conducted by self – administered questionnaire reported that 17 and 18% of respondents indicated that if they were to start again, they may not choose medicine as a career.[24] Neither study examined personal factors that might have predicted such feelings. A major long-term study entitled 'Medicine in Australia: Balancing Employment and Life' (MABEL)* has also looked at this issue and found that 85% of GPs and 87% of specialists are 'very' or 'moderately' satisfied with their work.[25]

Elsewhere, research has focussed on the minority of doctors who are unhappy or who perform at a substandard level professionally. This research tries to identify individuals who might have been better advised to enter some other career and more importantly seeks ways to better support distressed yet competent doctors so that they are not lost to the profession. In this book, the happy and successful doctors (the majority) might at times be seen to be overlooked but an honest emphasis on some negative aspects is necessary if you are to be accurately informed of what might lie ahead.

_____

* Other relevant reports from MABEL study can be found at https://melbourneinstitute.unimelb.edu.au/mabel/results-and-publications/reports-and-working-papers.

The UK group of over 1500 medical students mentioned above have been the subject of other follow up studies. One study used questionnaires to assess personality type, styles of approach to study and to work, and perceived workplace stress, with the aim of determining if any of these factors might correlate with career satisfaction.[26] Doctors who reported high job satisfaction were more likely to have a 'deep approach' to their work, and this approach correlated with a 'deep learning' style used at medical school. 'Deep learning' and a 'deep approach' to work were defined as an approach that sought understanding and integration of new material and was contrasted with a 'surface' approach, the latter implying studying for fear of failure, reading without understanding and not being well-organised. Satisfaction with medicine also correlated with the personality traits of greater extraversion and lower neuroticism.* Doctors who were less satisfied with their careers were marked by greater stress and emotional exhaustion, had higher neuroticism scores and were more likely to take a 'surface disorganised'† approach to work.

This study also found that many doctors reported 'high levels of personal accomplishment, choice and independence in their work environment, satisfaction with medicine as a career, and intellectual and emotional satisfaction from their work'. The authors were very cautious in their conclusions and emphasised that their findings related to correlations in a large cohort of doctors and that care should be taken in attempting to use the findings in making predictions about any individual doctor. They also emphasised that neither personality type nor learning style should be seen as solely determining one's destiny, noting that introverts can learn to be confident public speakers, people can be taught to better organise themselves and that 'neuroticism may be beneficial if sublimated into a

---

* Neuroticism is a basic personality trait described in psychology as an enduring tendency to experience negative emotional states. People who score highly for this trait are more likely to experience feelings of guilt, anxiety or depression and to respond less well to environmental stress.

† 'Surface-disorganised' as used by the authors included feelings of being overwhelmed by work, unsure of what was required and finding it difficult to organise time effectively.

professional concern for detail in critical situations, rather than merely being undifferentiated personal anxiety'.

These authors also commented on previous reports that suggested that doctors might be unhappy in their work because of the stressful work environment which included high workloads, lack of support and other perceived stresses. They pointed out that in their study the satisfied doctors were working in the same environment as the unhappy ones and suggested instead that burnout[*] in the medical workplace might be more a feature of the doctor's personality than the actual work environment. Doctors who are unhappy in their work are also likely to attribute some or all of their unhappiness to changes in the practice of medicine since the time that they graduated and will refer to over-regulation, increasing paper work, threats of being sued and diminished monetary rewards.

This is not to say that the working environment and workloads should be ignored. Indeed, it is likely that all doctors will eventually burn out if overworked for too long and especially if overwork is concurrent with one or more life crises such as bereavement or separation. Rather, it is to suggest that some of the normal pressures of a standard working environment for doctors can lead to stress and burnout in a proportion of predisposed doctors, unless those doctors are made aware of the risk and are taught better approaches to work, and to living, that can make them more secure, contented and resilient.

A 2007 study of 421 Norwegian medical students surveyed at the start, middle and end of a six-year course found that stress levels were higher in female students and that stress levels correlated with the traits of neuroticism and conscientiousness. The authors suggested that combinations of personality traits can predict stress at medical school.[27] If this is so, understanding your own personality and seeking advice and support when appropriate may help you cope better with challenging medical experiences at medical school. Approaches that might reduce stress and burnout (in medical students and in doctors) are discussed later.

---

[*] Burnout is said to have three components – emotional exhaustion, depersonalisation and reduced sense of personal accomplishment.

In addition to burnout and stress, anxiety and depression can also affect medical students; this is discussed in Section 4. It needs to be emphasised again that most doctors are content in their work and their lives, and so too are most medical students. For the minority of students and doctors who experience difficulties, the critical issue is to be aware that help is available and should be sought. Unfortunately, even though help is available, many students and doctors do not seek help, for a variety of reasons including denial, concern about stigmatisation, and a cultural attitude among members of the medical profession that doctors do not get sick or are not allowed to get sick.

1.10 I am interested in working in health care but perhaps not as a doctor. What other careers should I consider?

You have a number of options. Some young people feel attracted to work in health care but are concerned about seeking to enrol in medicine, perhaps because of the duration and cost of training, perhaps because they are not sure that being a doctor is right for them, or for other reasons. There is a wide range of university qualifications needed for the health care system and many of these career paths can lead to working independently of the hospital system. Most provide direct involvement in the care of patients and also provide very satisfying work. An incomplete list includes nurse, nurse practitioner, midwife, pharmacist, physiotherapist, paramedic, occupational therapist, clinical psychologist, dentist, dietician, optometrist, radiographer, speech therapist and social worker. All these professions approach their roles and work in a manner very similar to the medical profession, with high standards of training, expectations of continuing professional development and codes of ethical and professional conduct.

If you are uncertain or ambivalent about choosing medicine over any other area of health care, you should note that many entrants into graduate medical courses have originally graduated and worked in fields such as nursing or pharmacy. Thus taking such a pathway will not preclude a later career change and may bring benefits, including greater financial resources when you begin your four year medical course, deeper insights into our health care system and a qualification that provides opportunities for relevant part-time employment during your medical course.

THE MEDICAL SCHOOLS AND THE UNIVERSITY SELECTION PROCESSES

In this section I first provide information about the medical schools in Australia and explain the processes used by these schools to select students. This is followed by suggestions for preparing yourself for these selection processes and an examination of the cost of medical education and sources of financial support.

2.1 Where are the Australian medical schools located?

As at 2019, there were twenty-one accredited medical schools spread across all the states and territories of Australia.* The schools vary in size and together enrol approximately 3,800 new students each year.[1] As shown in the Table below, nine medical schools conduct school-leaver entry courses of five or six years duration (undergraduate or UG courses, accounting for approximately 1,400 places) while thirteen conduct graduate entry (GE) courses of four years duration (accounting for approximately 2,400 places).† Most of the

---

* The Northern Territory does not yet have an independent medical school but its clinical school is linked to Flinders University in Adelaide.

† Monash University conducts both a small GE and a larger UG course.

medical schools accept international medical students and of the 3,800 places available in Australia each year, approximately 650 are taken up by international students.[2]

Table 1: Australian medical schools

Undergraduate entry courses[*]	Graduate entry courses[†]
Bond University (five years)	Australian National University (four years)
Curtin University (five years)	Deakin University (four years)
James Cook University (six years)	Flinders University (four years)
Monash University UG (five years)	Griffith University (four years)
University of Adelaide (six years)	Macquarie University (four years)
University of Newcastle / University of New England (five years)	Monash University GE (four years)
University of New South Wales (six years)	University of Melbourne (four years)
University of Tasmania (five years)	University of Notre Dame Australia, Fremantle (four years)
Western Sydney University (five years)	University of Notre Dame Australia, Sydney (four years)
	University of Queensland (four years)
	University of Sydney (four years)

---

* Although the emphasis is on undergraduate entry (i.e. direct from year 12 at secondary school) some of these medical schools may also accept graduate entrants and internal transfers from another university course.

† With the exceptions of Flinders, Monash and Sydney Universities, these graduate entry medical schools form the GAMSAT Consortium and run a centralised entry process known as the Graduate Entry Medical School Admissions System (GEMSAS) to be found at http://www.gemsas.edu.au/.

	University of Western Australia (four years)
	University of Wollongong (four years)

The majority of the medical schools are in public universities where most student places are government supported. The medical school at Bond University on the Gold Coast in Queensland (a private institution) and the medical school at Macquarie University in Sydney offer only fee-paying places. The University of Notre Dame Australia, which has two medical schools, one in Sydney and one in Fremantle, has places that are government supported, and also offers full fee-paying places to Australian applicants.

To enable graduates to be registered to practise medicine, each medical course must be accredited by the Australian Medical Council (AMC). Accreditation is a rigorous process and accreditation must be maintained. The process is explained on the Council's website[3] where the accreditation reports for all medical courses can be found. Through the accreditation process all prospective students can be reassured about the quality of the education and training they will receive in Australia.

As mentioned in the introduction, the Australian Medical Students Association (AMSA), which is supported by the Australian Medical Association and many other organisations, maintains a helpful website (www.amsa.org.au) which includes a medical course guide with information about each course as provided by the universities as well as some commentaries from current students.[4] The AMSA site also gives other helpful advice to prospective students.

2.2 What is the difference between the graduate entry courses and the undergraduate courses? How long are the medical courses?

Graduate entry (GE) medical courses only accept people who have completed another university degree (their 'undergraduate' degree) so if you opt for this path, you will take a minimum of three years after completing year 12 at high school before you enter a medical course. At most GE courses, your first university degree can be in any field of study but the majority of prospective students choose science-related degrees or a course focussed on biomedical sciences[*] as offered by the university and recommended by the medical course. For example the GE course at the University of Melbourne requires that applicants must first complete an undergraduate degree with prerequisite studies in anatomy, physiology and biochemistry at second-year level (or equivalent).

GE courses are all of four years duration whereas UG courses are of five- or six-years duration. The GE option has advantages and disadvantages. One advantage is that the three years after you leave school will give you time to gain more experience of life. It will also give you time to think more about whether medicine is your preferred career choice. A disadvantage is that for those who have firmly made up their mind about getting into medical school then these might be seen as wasted years. In addition, there may be financial disadvantages through having to undertake two university courses.

For the medical schools that continue to enrol school leavers (undergraduate or UG courses), the learning experience will in general be very similar to the GE courses with the exception that the full time to complete the course is usually five or six years in duration, compared with four years for the GE courses. One potential disadvantage to consider is that if part way through the UG course you decide you do not wish

---

[*] Some students choose an undergraduate degree that leads to a professional role in the field of health as this may provide a better opportunity for part-time employment during the GE course.

to practise medicine, depending on how much of the course has been completed, your education may not have equipped you for much else. Some UG courses offer a Bachelor of Medical Sciences or similar degree which may include credit for subjects studied in the first sections of the medical course. A potential advantage is that if you apply initially for a UG course but miss out, you are still free to prepare and compete for a GE course.

As an examination of the websites of the medical schools will readily reveal, most courses have more than one pathway of entry. If you are planning to first pursue an UG course, you will be wise to think ahead about what your options are should you not be accepted. If this happens, and you wish to next apply for entry to a graduate course, considerable care needs to be taken in choosing your prior undergraduate degree. Some universities reserve a quota of places in their GE medical course for students who undertake their first degree at the same university, provided progress is satisfactory. As will be emphasised again later, careful study of the websites of the medical school or schools that you have in your sights is therefore essential.

2.3 Are these differences in the courses likely to be important to me?

For some students, factors such as geography ('I live near the university') or being determined to commence training as soon as possible will be strong influences on the choice of medical school – and that approach is quite reasonable. However, for others the differences might be important. For example, if your year 12 grades were not quite high enough to qualify for entry or if you have not done a particular prerequisite subject at high school, then the graduate entry courses give you another chance to enrol. If you are considering enrolling as a 'mature age' student (e.g. you have already studied and worked in another field such as education, nursing or pharmacy), graduate entry is probably the more realistic option for you.

Taking on a GE course a little later in your life means you are more likely to have a spouse/partner and/or children whose needs may influence your capacity to meet the requirements of the course or make meeting these requirements more stressful, so this might be worth thinking about. The pressures on married medical students are discussed in Section 3.6.

One Australian study comparing GE and UG courses found that the stresses experienced in the medical course differed, with UG entrants expressing more doubts about their career choice while GE entrants reported more concerns about study/work commitment balance.[5] This may be more a reflection of the age of the students than differences between the two types of courses. A more recent study, based on questionnaire responses, found little differences between the students enrolled at UG and GE courses and noted that the groups were equally satisfied with the choice of course they had made. No differences were observed in regard to self-reported coping or burnout. However, UG entrants scored higher on empathy levels while GE entrants reported higher levels of alcohol use and hazardous drinking.[6]

There are no data to indicate that the type of course (graduate entry or undergraduate) has a significant influence on the characteristics or performance of graduates, or any influence on career path options after the intern year, so the issue of your future career path plans should not be taken strongly into your considerations in making your decision about a preferred medical course. Medical Deans Australia and New Zealand commenced a long-term study in 2004 entitled the 'Medical Schools Outcomes Database' which is designed to track medical graduates into prevocational and vocational training* and assess the outcomes of educational programs. In time, information from this study may be very helpful to you in making decisions about where to study medicine.[7]

---

* The period of further medical training after graduation from medical school is divided into an initial general phase (prevocational training) followed by dedicated training in general practice or another specialty (vocational training) as described in more detail in Section 5.

2.4 Are there any other differences between the courses?

There are some other aspects of the medical courses that could influence your choice. For example, if you are already intent on a career that will involve practice in rural Australia, you should consider which medical courses provide the strongest rural medicine educational experience. If you sense that part, or all, of your career will be focussed on medical research, then you may wish to choose a medical course that places greater emphasis on research. If you are an Indigenous Australian, you are likely to be interested in the culture of the medical course and its history of support for Indigenous students.[8]

You may also wish to consider the learning/teaching methods employed in any medical course and the resources available to support student learning. In the Australian Medical Education Study (AMES), commissioned by the Federal Government in 2005,[9] interns surveyed felt that the methods of learning and teaching (specifically problem-based learning* versus more traditional education) used in their medical course impacted on some aspects of their preparedness for the intern year. This finding supports an earlier Australian study.[10] This issue is discussed further in Sections 3.2, 3.3 and 5.1.

You may be puzzled by the different titles given to medical graduates of our universities as these now include MB, BS (Bachelor of Medicine and Bachelor of Surgery) and MD (Doctor of Medicine) as well as combined degrees such as Bachelor of Medical Science and Doctor of Medicine or Bachelor of Clinical Science and Doctor of Medicine. These differences in title can generally be ignored as all courses are required as part of their accreditation by the Australian Medical Council to have a program that will adequately prepare their graduates for the intern year. Thus the different titles are of no significance when you graduate, seek to be registered with the Medical Board of Australia and commence an internship. They should be regarded primarily as marketing devices by which each medical school

---

* Problem-based learning is discussed in more detail on page 80.

seeks to distinguish itself. To be entitled to award the MD (a postgraduate degree), the medical course must have an additional component of research to meet the Master's level (Level 9) set down under the Australian Qualifications Framework.

Studies have indicated that there may be differences between medical courses as to how well-prepared graduates feel for the intern experience. Courses that offer 'early, structured and sustained' clinical experience seem to do better in this regard.[11] Another factor that may be important to consider is the size of the medical school and the cohesiveness of the student groups with whom you will learn. In those medical schools with large enrolments, you may want to examine how students are allocated to subgroups. Ideally a large enrolment needs to be divided into smaller clinical schools,* with each school being the home base for each group of students for their entire clinical training.

Some medical courses are widely dispersed such that clinical rotations between cities, towns and even states may be encountered. These rotations may not be optional. Such rotations might be rewarding and unproblematic for a single student but may be unsettling and disruptive for those with partners who have their own careers. Where clinical schools are widely dispersed, the cost of accommodation may be an issue and transport may be problematic so that having a car and a driving licence may be essential. For students who need to maintain part time work to support themselves, distant rotations might also be problematic.

The federal government has encouraged and funded universities to establish clinical schools in rural areas to train more doctors who will eventually work in rural medical practice. These rural clinical schools are now well-established and have proven effective[12] and popular with students.[13]

Most medical schools offer and expect students to undertake an elective term during the latter part of the course to experience medicine in a

---

* A clinical school refers to an independent sub-section of the medical school housed in its own building and usually located in a major public hospital in a city or in the case of rural clinical schools, in a rural hospital.

completely different environment. Elective terms can be spent in Australia or overseas. The latter option may be difficult for students who are married, have children or cannot afford to travel. Students generally enjoy and value their elective wherever it is spent.

2.5 Tell me some more about each Australian medical school*

Detailed information about each medical school and its university is available at the relevant websites. A brief summary of information drawn from those websites is attached at the end of this section. The medical schools are listed alphabetically. For each medical school, the total number of student places available is provided. The total number for each school includes government supported places and bonded places, as well as places set aside for selected groups (e.g. Indigenous students or students with rural backgrounds). As a prospective student, you are strongly advised to carefully read all the information available on the websites of those medical schools under consideration. The layout and flow of information on each website varies considerably and it may take some time to find all the information you are seeking. The AMSA website may also be consulted.[14]

Almost all the medical schools accept applications from international applicants as well as from domestic applicants. 'Domestic' applicants include Australian and New Zealand citizens, Australian permanent residents (but not NZ permanent residents) and holders of an Australian humanitarian visa. International applicants to GE medical schools will be required to provide a GAMSAT score (see below) or a score from the North American equivalent, the Medical Colleges Admission Test (MCAT). International applicants whose education has not been in English will be required to meet an English language standard.† All successful international applicants

---

* Every effort has been made to accurately summarise the information available on the website of each medical school but the author advises the reader to make their own assessment of the original source.

† It should be noted that whether one's medical degree was obtained in Australia

will pay full tuition fees, the details of which are available on the relevant medical school website. International students who complete their medical course in Australia are not guaranteed an intern position, which is essential for progression to full medical registration with the Medical Board of Australia (see also Section 5).

If your application is successful, admission to a medical course will require provision of proof of an undergraduate degree (for GE courses) and may require provision of a police check and a first aid certificate.[15] Clinical placements may have other requirements such as working with children checks, health and safety induction, and hand hygiene instruction. Each medical school will require conformity with its infectious diseases and immunisation policies (see Section 4.8). All medical students in Australia are required to be registered with the Medical Board of Australia via the Australian Health Practitioner Regulation Agency (AHPRA). Registration is free and is handled by each university on behalf of the student. For the vast majority of students this is unproblematic. However for students with a record of a criminal conviction, this may be a barrier to registration, if not as a medical student then later at the point of graduation and registration as a doctor. AHPRA and the Medical Board of Australia have to heed the national law on this matter. Section 58 (headed 'Unsuitability to hold general registration') of the national law in para (1) (b) reads as follows an

(1) A National Board may decide an individual is not a suitable person to hold general registration in a health profession if –

(b) having regard to the individual's criminal history to the extent that is relevant to the individual's practice of the profession, the individual is not, in the Board's opinion, an appropriate person to practise the profession or it is not in the public interest for the individual to practise the profession;

Certain disabilities may also need to be considered by applicants

via a UG course or a GE course, the medical registration process with the Medical Board of Australia also has an English language standard to be met.

to medical school as some disabilities may be sufficiently limiting as to prevent registration for clinical practice. This is discussed in more detail in Section 2.14.

For many prospective medical students, finding suitable and affordable accommodation at or near the university will be an important consideration. Most universities employ housing officers to assist students to find accommodation and many have halls of residence or other styles of accommodation on campus. More information can be found on the university websites.

In examining any website, prospective students should pay attention to whether the medical school offers its own scholarships or bursaries, in addition to the financial support available via government (see Section 2.20).

2.6 How difficult is it to get into medical school?

Entry to a medical course is highly competitive and the number of applicants is much greater than the number of places available. The change to graduate entry at some medical schools increased the number of applicants to the continuing undergraduate courses in Australia such that there are now at least ten applicants for each student place.[16] This development has also resulted in many more students making multiple applications, including to medical schools in states other than their own. You will need to think through your intentions and consider all the implications of applying for and then accepting a place at a medical school in another state or territory. The timing and process of applying for medical school is described below in Section 2.12.

The implications commence with the cost of travelling interstate if you are offered one or more interviews. If your application is successful, you will need to think about how you will adjust to living in a new city, perhaps away from home for the first time; how easily you feel you will be able to create a new circle of friends or take up your usual leisure activities;

and what financial issues might arise. Once enrolled in a medical course, it can be very difficult to transfer to a course in your home state even on compassionate grounds. In the longer term, a decision to study medicine in another state may well result in your making that state your permanent home.

Second or third round offers of places are not uncommon and may sometimes be made even after the academic year has begun, so a degree of flexibility and a willingness to move at short notice is required.[17]

2.7 On what basis are selections made?

The selection of young people to train to become doctors has been the subject of much thought and discussion, increasing research, and considerable change over the last twenty years in Australia and also in many other countries. Previously applicants were selected solely on their year 12 final examination performance. Now there is general agreement (in Australia) that the selection process should aim to choose people with the cognitive (academic) abilities and other non-academic, personal or non-cognitive* qualities to be able to cope with a long, demanding and potentially stressful course and to select people who have the potential to become 'good doctors'. The best predictors of success in the medical course are held to be prior academic performance, English language skills and reading ability.[18]

The discussions about selection have especially focused on the notion that assessment of the humanistic, non-academic qualities of prospective doctors should be a part of the process. The methods used to assess non-cognitive qualities and attributes include (a) components of the University Clinical Aptitude Test (UCAT) and GAMSAT national testing procedures as described below, (b) interview and (c) for a small number of medical courses, provision of a personal portfolio or written statement. In addition, some universities use an online test designed to assess a range of personal

_____
* Non-cognitive, personal or non-academic qualities are explained in Section 1.2

qualities that are considered to be important for the study and practice of medicine known as personal qualities assessment (PQA). There is continuing debate (and research) into the value of assessing non-academic attributes, especially for undergraduate applicants for entrance.[19]

Selection into undergraduate entry courses is for most courses based on a combination of school performance (ATAR), UCAT score and interview. Specific information about selection criteria and any prerequisite requirements can be found on each school website (see also section 2.13).

Selection into graduate entry medicine is based on up to four criteria: GAMSAT score, grade point average* (GPA), performance in interview and scoring of a portfolio or special application or supplementary form or personal statement. The way in which each university combines these criteria when making their final offers varies.[†]

The selection procedures in Australia are intended to be equitable, consistent and transparent. These principles about selection and the procedures discussed above are generally agreed. There is evidence that each selection criterion predicts success in different aspects of the medical course.[20] For example in a 2016 report, it was found that at one GE course the GAMSAT score correlated best with performance in years 1 and 2, the interview score predicted performance in the clinical years 3 and 4 and the GPA predicted performance across all 4 years.[21] However, there is little evidence available to date that the selection methods achieve their ultimate intention, viz. to choose applicants who will become competent, caring and contented 'good' doctors when they enter independent practice.[22]

While most medical schools combine the year 12 academic results (for UG entry) or grade point averages (for GE courses) with scores on a nationwide examination (UCAT for UG courses and GAMSAT for GE courses – see below) and assessment by interview, there remains considerable variation as to the weight placed on these three measures. There is also

---

* The grade point average is the average result of all your grades in your undergraduate degree and is calculated on a 7-point grading scale, with 7 being the highest and 0 the lowest (fail).

† More information about selection for the majority of GE schools is available at http://www.gemsas.edu.au/.

variation in the purpose and format of the interview. A small number of medical schools also require the submission of a personal portfolio (see below) that is subjected to a formal rating process and added to these assessment tools. Several medical schools have alternative entry paths for Indigenous students that do not use UMAT or GAMSAT. These variations mean that it is essential that you carefully examine the requirements of each institution to which you are considering applying.

2.8 What are UCAT, GAMSAT and ISAT?

UCAT and GAMSAT are national entry/aptitude tests used for entry to nearly all Australian medical schools. ISAT is a test of intellectual skills and abilities available for international students.

UCAT is the University Clinical Aptitude Test and is based on a similar test that has been used for school-leaver entry to medical school in the UK for more than ten years.[23] It has been developed for use by a consortium of Australian and New Zealand universities that conduct undergraduate entry medical schools. The test is delivered by a commercial company, Pearson Vue, on set dates at a range of sites throughout Australia, New Zealand and at some overseas locations. It is an online test that takes two hours to complete and has five sections covering verbal reasoning, decision making, quantitative reasoning, abstract reasoning and situational judgement.[24]

UCAT is not based on any prior learning or on the school curriculum and there are no prerequisite subjects. However candidates are strongly advised to use the free official practice tests and other helpful information on the UCAT website to prepare for the test and to familiarise themselves with the format and timing (www.ucat.edu.au). As occurred with the predecessor Undergraduate Medicine and Health Sciences Admission Test (UMAT), it is likely that commercial preparation courses will be marketed. A 2012 UK study based on a questionnaire response from a large number of UCAT candidates indicated that students who put more time into preparation scored better, particularly those who had used the free official practice tests and a second source of preparation, including for some a commercial course.[25] Candidates who had studied a higher level of mathematics also scored better, both overall and in the quantitative reasoning segment. Of concern, this study also suggested that students from less well-resourced schools did not perform as well as others.

A 2013 Australian study[26] (based on the previous UMAT and not the UCAT) also indicated that commercial coaching improved scores but only for Section 3 on non-verbal reasoning. Coaching had no benefit for Section 2 on understanding people and may have led to worse scores in Section 1 on logical reasoning. The benefit of coaching for Section 3 was only apparent for students of high academic ability. The study also showed that students attending selective high schools performed better, even after controlling for academic ability. The authors suggested that these findings related to these students spending more time on practising and that coaching alone without sustained practice is unlikely to bring improved results.

There are strict rules regarding who may sit the UCAT. It cannot be taken until a candidate is in their final year of secondary schooling. It can also be taken by candidates during or after completion of an undergraduate degree but such candidates may not be offered a place in an undergraduate medical course. Each medical school website will provide relevant information. Some undergraduate medical schools require international students to sit the UCAT and again each school's website needs to be consulted for this detail.

The Graduate Australian Medical School Admissions Test (GAMSAT) was first used in 1996. It was developed by the Australian Council of Educational Research on behalf of a consortium of graduate entry medical schools. Its purpose is to assess capacity to undertake high level intellectual studies in a demanding course. The test is divided into three discrete sections, one devoted to reasoning in humanities and social sciences, one to written communication and the third and biggest section to reasoning in biological and physical sciences. The test takes five and a half hours with a one-hour recess. No prerequisite subjects are identified, and the emphasis of the examination is on reasoning. However, the nature of the material covered in the section of GAMSAT covering reasoning in biological and physical sciences assumes year 12 level knowledge of physics and first year university level knowledge of biology and chemistry. An early study of the outcomes of GAMSAT demonstrated better performance by applicants who had completed science degrees. That study also confirmed that graduates with a background in arts and social sciences could be successful.[27]

Commercial courses are available to help students prepare for GAMSAT. Preparation for UCAT and GAMSAT is discussed further in Section 2.17.

The GAMSAT test is offered twice a year, in March and September. Only persons with a university degree or who are enrolled in the last year of a degree course are eligible to sit. The fee in 2019 for those sitting the test in Australia was $606. GAMSAT is held on the same day in most Australian capital cities and in Townsville and is available in the Ireland, United Kingdom, United States of America, New Zealand and Singapore.

There are no limits to the number of times one can sit GAMSAT but the GE medical schools have a policy of only accepting a GAMSAT score from a test taken within two years of the date of the application to a GE course.[*]

The International Student Admissions Test (ISAT) was developed by the Australian Council of Educational Research.[28] It is a 3-hour computer-based multiple-choice test designed to assess a candidate's intellectual skills and abilities that are the foundation of academic success at tertiary level. ISAT is administered through thousands of Prometric Inc. centres around the world. There are no set dates for ISAT testing so candidates can register and sit at a time and place of their choosing. ISAT is not used by all Australian medical schools so international students must inform themselves about the requirements of any school under consideration.

_____

[*] More detailed information, including sample questions and a practice examination (for purchase) can be found at http://gamsat.acer.edu.au/.

2.9 What does an interview usually entail?

The nature and purpose of the interview varies between the medical schools. Some use a single interview by a panel usually composed of three people, including a doctor from the medical school, a doctor in independent practice and a community member. Others use a multi-station mini-interview[29] (MMI) where the applicant moves from station to station to respond to various set questions and scenarios and the interviewers have been trained for their role. MMIs are not standardised between medical schools as the questions and scenarios are typically linked to the aptitudes and qualities that any school is seeking. For example Monash University uses an MMI with eight separate stations and advises on its website that the scenarios and associated questions are intended to focus on an applicant's relevant personal qualities such as quality of motivation, appropriateness of style, communication skills, ability to work in a team, leadership, empathy, logical thinking and ability to function under pressure.

By comparison, the University of Notre Dame Australia, Fremantle, advises on its website that interviews will be conducted by trained teams including academic, general and community members and describes the interview as an opportunity for the applicant to demonstrate personal qualities such as communication skills, empathy and motivation. In some medical schools, the interview is used to 'deselect' unsuitable applicants, while others use a formal score, especially from the MMI, which is incorporated in an overall selection ranking score. The logistics of conducting interviews in a timely and cost-effective way has led to only a proportion of applicants being offered an interview. Pre-selection for interview is usually based on the UCAT or GAMSAT ranking.

Interestingly, a small pilot comparison study from a Canadian university indicated that students preferred the MMI to a traditional interview.[30] One argument in favour of the MMI is that poor performance at a single station is likely to have less impact on the interview score than poor handling of one question at a panel interview. Here in Australia there is anecdotal evidence that applicants undergoing panel interviews report a preference for its more personal approach as it provides an opportunity to establish rapport with interviewers over a longer period of time.[31] Preparation for interview is discussed below.

2.10 What should be in a personal portfolio?

Only a few medical schools require a written personal statement or portfolio. The University of Notre Dame Australia at Fremantle (which is explicitly trying to select students with a positive attitude to working in under-served communities) uses the personal statement to examine rural background, higher research degrees and research experience, work experience, sporting, music, church and other participation or leadership activities, experience working with charitable agencies or with underserved communities, and languages spoken other than English. The university asks for a curriculum vitae, two written references, and a personal statement about reasons for studying medicine. The University of Notre Dame Australia at Sydney uses the personal statement in a similar manner.

Wollongong University advises that the portfolio allows students to highlight areas of achievement, leadership, teamwork, service ethic and commitment, and ties to regional, rural or remote areas. The medical school website provides a template for constructing a portfolio with detailed advice and guidance as to what is being sought.[32]

2.11 Are there any other factors taken into consideration?

These assessment processes are not the only factors that influence selection. Most medical schools reserve places for Indigenous applicants and as described above some use alternative selection processes for Indigenous applicants. Most schools also reserve places for rural applicants.* In some

_____

* There is now a universally applicable definition of a rural applicant, viz. one who, as of 31 December in the year prior to degree commencement, has spent at least five medical schools adjustments are made to the scoring system to seek to ensure that students from less advantaged backgrounds are represented in each intake. The selection processes for overseas fee paying students may differ again.

2.12 When does selection take place and how, when and where do I apply?

There are two (and in some states three) phases to making an application. The first phase is to apply to sit the UCAT or the GAMSAT. The second phase is to apply to one or more of the medical schools of your choice. Apart from the centralised Graduate Entry Medical School Admissions System (GEMSAS) system for most of the GE medical schools as described below, the requirements for application vary. The timelines of each medical school are strictly enforced and it is the applicant's responsibility not to miss any deadline.

For UG entry schools the timing of the dates for initial application and of interview, for those selected, is at the discretion of each medical school so each web site needs to be carefully inspected. In some states, entry to all undergraduate courses, including medicine, is coordinated via a central state office known most commonly as a tertiary admissions scheme. Information about these schemes is available on each medical school website.

For GE schools, the GAMSAT consortium has developed a centralised application system known as GEMSAS.* This guide provides

---

consecutive years, or 10 years cumulatively, in an Australian Standard Geographic Classification – Remoteness Areas (ASGCRA) RA 2-5 area, from birth (i.e. during any period in their life) is eligible to apply under the Rural Background entry pathway. The time frame is based on the location of your primary residence. For guidance on Remoteness Area locations (RA) please visit the website below and use the search tool at Remoteness Area Location (RA): http://www.doctorconnect.gov. au/internet/otd/publishing.nsf/Content/ra-intro.

* The system's guide for admission to graduate medicine can be found at http:// www.gemsas.edu.au/.

more information about the precise selection criteria of each participating medical school. The guide also covers such matters as the number of places available and their sources of funding, the necessary GAMSAT score or GPA to be a realistic candidate at each course, dates for information sessions and the availability of scholarships. It helpfully lists all the universities that participate in the automated results transfer system (ARTS).

In 2019 GEMSAS applications for domestic students (to commence medicine in 2020) opened on 30 April and closed on 31 May. The system matches applicants to a single interview at their highest preferred medical school where they are ranked within the interview quota. Interviews are usually conducted in late September. Applicants interviewed at any participating medical school who are not offered a place at that school are automatically considered for admission at a lower preference medical school.* Standardised interview scores are fed into the online system and applicants are matched to their highest preferred medical school where they are ranked within the selection quota. It is important to note that Flinders University, Monash University and the University of Sydney do not participate in GEMSAS and the medical school websites of those three universities need to be consulted individually.

2.13 Are there any prerequisites?

Most but not all the UG medical schools list one or two secondary school subjects as recommended or as required subjects, most often chemistry. Some also mention the need for adequate skills in English. Each medical school's website should be consulted. Prospective students with disabilities should read Sections 2.14 and 3.7 and seek information from the medical schools.

---

* All participating medical schools conduct interviews, some by a single panel and the others by MMI. The GEMSAS website states: 'Interview scores for each applicant are standardised to give a score that can be used by other participating schools in the allocations for offers of places. In practice, applicants will have the best chance of an offer from the school where they were interviewed.' How this standardisation is done is not explained and thus it is difficult to give advice regarding how to list your preferred medical schools.

The GE medical schools (with the exception of the University of Melbourne and Macquarie University and in the near future, the University of Queensland) do not have any prerequisite subjects, but as their name indicates, applicants must (by the time they are accepted) have completed an UG degree. While the GE schools have a general policy of encouraging and welcoming applicants who have completed a humanities degree, and, while such applicants have been successful, the majority of successful applicants have completed a science or health (e.g. nursing, pharmacy or physiotherapy) degree. This may be because science subjects are more attractive to potential medical students but probably also reflects the requirements of the reasoning in biological and physical sciences component of the GAMSAT.

2.14 Can persons with disabilities consider studying medicine?

People with disabilities are protected by law from discrimination. Therefore, based on first principles there should be little to prevent a disabled student who has been selected to study medicine by the selection processes outlined above from starting and completing the medical course. However, there are some practical issues during the course and some registration issues after graduation that need to be objectively considered.

The medical course will involve not only acquiring knowledge from lectures, tutorials, books and other sources but also learning physical skills such as physically examining patients and learning minor procedures (measuring blood pressure, taking blood samples etc.). These physical tasks require some manual dexterity as well as good eyesight and adequate hearing. Thus some physical disabilities might hamper a student's progress. Such limitations might also prevent a disabled student from completing all the requirements of the intern year, even though those same disabilities may not be relevant to a range of career possibilities beyond the intern year. Students with disabilities should look at the medical school websites for information and seek advice from the relevant medical faculty.

Most medical school websites refer to detailed guidelines prepared by Medical Deans Australia New Zealand that describe the inherent requirements of the medical course.[33] In preparing these guidelines the medical deans sought to balance the provision of the greatest possible access for students with a disability, consistent with national disability discrimination law, while ensuring safe clinical training and having regard to the eventual requirements for registration as an intern with the Medical Board of Australia. The guidelines are not mandatory and their application may vary between medical schools. Disabled students will be wise to read this document in preparation for a discussion with staff at the medical school of their choosing. Doing so should permit a realistic self-assessment as to whether clinical medicine is the right career to choose.

Depending upon the advice received from a medical school, advice may also be needed from the state agency (postgraduate medical council – see Section 5.2) that accredits intern training positions. Advice may also be needed from the AHPRA and the Medical Board of Australia about the statutory requirements that have to be met for provisional medical registration (see also page 94).

Another form of disability is the carriage of a transmissible illness that might be spread to patients. A small proportion of medical students may be asymptomatic ('healthy') carriers of viral infections such as hepatitis B, hepatitis C or HIV. Depending upon the degree of 'infectivity' as assessed by laboratory testing, carriers may be excluded from undertaking certain medical and surgical procedures because of the risk of accidentally transmitting the infection to a patient. This still leaves a wide range of clinical practice open to the graduate but will require approval of a slightly modified intern training program. This issue is discussed in more detail in Section 4.8.

Although not necessarily a disability, some chronic relapsing illnesses that can afflict young people (e.g. Crohn's disease, some mental disorders such as bipolar disorder or recurrent depression) might make it more difficult to complete a demanding medical course. If you are in such a category, you should take advice from your treating doctor and keep in contact with your doctor during the course.

Students with learning disorders such as dyslexia or information processing difficulties, who have been able to cope at school through being allowed additional time to complete assessments and examinations, may find the demands of clinical medicine very challenging.

As mentioned earlier, all prospective students need to carefully consider if they will be able to cope with a demanding course and with subsequent clinical practice which can be burdensome. This advice applies even more so to prospective students with disabilities, whether these disabilities are physical or non-physical.

2.15 What if I am not an Australian or New Zealand citizen or Australian resident? Can I apply from another country?

Yes, most Australian medical schools set aside places in the course for students from other countries. These students are expected to pay the full cost of that tuition. The costs vary between medical schools and will change over time so the university websites should be looked at for this detail. The selection processes also vary between the medical schools and again each medical school's website should be inspected. One feature in common between all medical schools is that the assessment of applicants from other countries will include a requirement that applicants take the UCAT or GAMSAT or an equivalent entry test.* As discussed above, UCAT and GAMSAT are held once each year in a small number of cities in other countries. For students who are considering an undergraduate entry medical course, there may be advantages (in terms of adjusting to a different culture, improving English language skills and preparing for UCAT) in coming to Australia for the last one or two years of high school.

If you are from outside Australia and New Zealand and have only just begun to think about applying to study medicine here, you may also want

---

* The North American Medical Colleges Admissions Test (MCAT) is an acceptable alternative for most Australian GE schools. MCAT is held in many cities around the world, see http://www.aamc.org/students/applying/mcat.

to read more generally about the Australian education system and about life and the cost of living here.*

An important consideration if you are coming from another country is access to the experience of the intern year. As described elsewhere, the intern year is compulsory for meeting Australian requirements for full medical registration. Access to intern training positions in Australia is influenced by the availability of training places and by federal government migration and visa policies.[34] International medical students are not guaranteed an intern position. Applicants from other countries should explore whether an Australian medical degree will permit them to undertake an intern or pre-registration year in their country of origin or elsewhere. Most Australian medical school websites provide links to official guidance about this aspect.

International students also need to be aware that two Australian universities have established AMC-accredited medical courses partly based in other countries (Monash University in Malaysia and the University of Queensland in New Orleans in the USA).

2.16 What if English is not my first language?

There is a community expectation and a legislated requirement for medical registration that doctors in Australia be reasonably fluent in spoken English and competent in written English. The English language standards expected by Australian medical schools are usually readily found on the relevant website. Most universities offer bridging courses to international students to enhance their language skills. Advanced English language skills are needed to maximise the learning opportunities in the medical course and for the successful completion of the course. The Medical Board of Australia has published its English language skills 'registration standard'.[35] The standard is set at IELTS academic level 7.[36] These standards do not have to be met for student registration (see page 92) but are compulsory for

---

* Useful information can be found at this website: https://www.studyinaustralia. gov.au/.

registration for the intern year. In practice, the standard required for entry into an Australian medical course is usually the same as that required by the Medical Board.

2.17 How can I prepare for the selection processes?
Preparing for UCAT or GAMSAT

Medical school selection is highly competitive and it is essential that you have a good understanding of the composition of the UCAT or GAMSAT before you sit. You should carefully review the sample questions and answers available at the relevant website. The advice offered on behalf of the two consortia of medical schools which commissioned the UCAT and GAMSAT is that no special training or coaching is needed for either test. However, commercial organisations in Australia now offer coaching for admission to a medical school and many students avail themselves of these services.

The section of GAMSAT dealing with reasoning in biological and physical sciences assumes a year 12 level of knowledge of physics and a first-year university level of knowledge of biology and chemistry. If your selection of subjects at high school and/or your undergraduate course has not given you sufficient exposure to these subjects, then you should seek advice about how to best prepare yourself.

An Australian study examined the effect of coaching for both the UMAT (the test that preceded the UCAT) and interview (multi-station mini interview) in 287 applicants selected for interview at an undergraduate entry medical course.[37] In the study, half the 287 participants said they had sought coaching for UMAT. When UMAT scores were examined, there were no significant differences between the coached and non-coached groups for the components of tests of logical reasoning or understanding people but the coached students performed better on the tests of non-verbal reasoning. The results of this study about coaching for interview are discussed below. Whether these findings can be extrapolated to the new UCAT is unknown. A later New Zealand study showed no benefit in UMAT scores but did note that participation in preparatory courses made students feel more confident of success.[38] In addition this was not a prospective randomised study and thus the findings must be viewed cautiously.

A survey in 2008 of first year students in the graduate entry course at the University of Sydney gained responses from 43% of students, of whom just under half had undertaken some form of coaching, either for GAMSAT or the MMI or both. The mean GAMSAT score for the group who received coaching was a little lower than for those who had no coaching while the opposite was true for the scores for the MMI. The authors concluded that coaching offered little advantage.[39]

A review of studies on the effect of commercial courses on results in the Medical College Admission Test (used in the USA and Canada for entry to medical school) concluded that the utility and value of these courses had not been demonstrated.[40] The authors suggested that student anxiety and aggressive marketing had allowed the courses to prosper.

Despite the absence of data to show that taking part in such commercial courses is of real benefit, successful applicants who participate in such courses are inclined to attribute their success to that investment of time and money.[41]

As there is no limit on the number of times that a university graduate may sit the GAMSAT, you may be tempted to sit again and again until you reach a score that gets you to an interview. Whether this is a wise idea after say four attempts only you can decide.

Preparing for interviews

As already noted, the nature of the interview varies from medical school to medical school as does the purpose of the interview and the use to which the interview 'results' are put. It is thus essential that you read carefully what each school website says about the nature, aims and conduct of any interview. The following advice is intended to help you at interview to come across as the person you really are. There is no point in your trying to 'second guess' the purpose of any questions asked at interview. Training to provide the 'right' answers to particular questions is not advised. However, you should participate in some practice interviews to reduce anxiety levels for the 'real thing', to think about predictable questions, and to help you feel fluent in explaining what it is that is attracting you to study medicine. In MMI interviews, you should seek to explain your thinking behind any answers that you give to questions as this will allow the interviewers to more readily appreciate your qualities. If you have the opportunity to take advice from students who have recently been through the interview process, this can also be helpful.

The Australian study mentioned above also examined the effect of coaching for MMI. In this group of 287 applicants, approximately half said they had received coaching. However, the coached group did no better in their overall MMI score and at one of the nine stations (the one testing communication skills) they did worse. Seventeen applicants participated in the MMI on two occasions and subgroup analysis showed an improved performance at the interview stations that used the same questions as at the previous year.[42] The candidates themselves felt that a practice run at an MMI would be helpful but considered coaching for interview the least useful aid to success.

You should also think about how to dress for an interview. Interviewers are instructed not to take personal appearance into account but you are more likely to make a favourable impression if you dress modestly and are well groomed, as would be expected of a professional person.

Preparing a portfolio

Only a small number of medical schools ask applicants to submit a personal portfolio. You should check the medical school's web site for what is expected and if possible examine a previously submitted portfolio or take advice from someone who is familiar with the requirement of that medical school. Further advice is provided in Section 2.10.

2.18 Is it possible to study medicine in another state?

Yes, there are no geographical constraints for making application to enter any medical school in Australia. Some medical schools have selection processes that are weighted in favour of local applicants (e.g. the University of Western Sydney medical school sets a slightly lower academic achievement score for applicants who have resided in the Greater Western Sydney region for five years). In addition, at several medical schools some of the supported and bonded places are reserved for local applicants.

As mentioned above, there are many implications of living and studying interstate for four or more years that you need to think about (see Section 2.6).

2.19 Can I go overseas for my medical course? And if so, will I be able to work in Australia?

Yes, a small number of Australian citizens who have been unsuccessful in obtaining a place in an Australian medical course have moved to other countries to undertake medical training. There are cost implications which are not addressed here. After completion of the course, you may be required to undergo further assessment in Australia before the overseas qualification is recognised and before you are able to obtain medical registration. You may be required to sit the examinations of the Australian Medical Council designed for international medical graduates, and/or obtain the equivalent of a supervised intern year position before you can be granted full registration. These requirements vary according to the country in which the degree was obtained. More information is available on the websites of the Australian Medical Council and the Medical Board of Australia.

2.20 How much do medical courses cost in Australia? Are scholarships or other support schemes available?

Medical education is expensive. However, for most domestic students, the cost is heavily subsidised by the Federal Government through what are called Commonwealth Supported Places (CSP). Receipt of CSP does not cover the full cost of a medical course and involves a student contribution to the cost of their education. The amount of this contribution is set by each university but is capped by law and in 2018 the maximum annual contribution that could be asked of a medical student was $10,596. Most Australian students are eligible for assistance in paying this fee via the HECS-HELP scheme (HECS standing for the Higher Education Contribution Scheme). This is a loan which has to be gradually re-paid to the Australian Tax Office (ATO) after graduation and when earning above a level of income set by the government via the ATO. The amount of debt is indexed (meaning that the debt owed is adjusted regularly in line with the consumer price index). There are very strict regulations and time limits for applications for CSP and HECS-HELP that must be observed. These places are only available to Australian citizens and permanent residents, and New Zealand citizens and permanent residents. Note that CSP does not contribute to meeting accommodation and daily living expenses.[43]

A fixed proportion (28.5% in 2016) of Commonwealth Supported Places are also Bonded Medical Places (BMP) such that, from 2020, recipients are obliged to work in an eligible location in Australia for a total of three years, with the three years of service to be completed within 18 years of graduation. These eligible locations are defined as those regarded as rural and remote or experiencing workforce shortages.[44] The three years of service needed to fulfil one's obligations is now flexible and can be undertaken as non-continuous full-time, part-time or even via fly in/fly out duties. The process of applying for or being offered a BMP is handled by the staff of each medical school. A decision to accept a BMP should be taken carefully as you will be signing a contract that will be expensive should you break it.

Some changes to the BMP scheme were made for 2020 and may have implications for current students and recent graduates participating in the scheme.*

There are other sources of financial support to study for a medical degree. The Australian Defence Force (ADF) offers well-funded scholarships that are bonded for the length of the period of the scholarship plus one year. ADF support can be applied for at any point before or during your medical course.†

A range of other more narrowly targeted scholarships and subsidies are available. These include the Bendigo and Adelaide Bank Scholarship for Rural and Regional Australians. This provides $5,000 per year for Australians living in rural/regional Australia who are attending university for the first time and studying full time.[45]

For students who need to relocate for their studies, financial support may be available in the form of the Centrelink Relocation Scholarship.[46] In addition, depending upon your financial circumstances and your age, you may be entitled to Youth Allowance, Austudy and Rent Assistance from Centrelink.‡

The John Flynn Placement Program[47] supports short placements of medical students in remote medical practices to foster medical student interest in remote and rural medicine. These placements are scheduled outside the normal weeks of any medical course program.

Individual medical schools may offer scholarships and bursaries restricted to their own students so each web site should be inspected. In addition, for enrolled students who later experience financial difficulties, support may be available from your university.

---

*   Transitional arrangements are in place for past recipients and details can be found at www.health.gov.au/bmpscheme.

†   More detail is available at http://www.defencejobs.gov.au/education/university-sponsorship/.

‡   To find out more about your eligibility or to make a claim see www.humanservices.gov.au. Information is also available at https://www.studyassist.gov.au/front.

2.21 Support for Indigenous Australians wishing to enter medicine

From having no Indigenous doctors a generation ago, in the last ten years the number has increased from around 150 to almost 400. However, this remains well below the number of Indigenous students that would be expected based on the proportion of the Australian population that is Indigenous. There is an active Indigenous doctors' association[48] which provides support for Indigenous medical students. Australia has a long way to go to match the performance of Canada, the USA and New Zealand in enrolling and retaining Indigenous medical students.

An early leader in the endeavour to increase Indigenous enrolment was the University of Newcastle which has produced over 100 Indigenous medical graduates and maintains an active program.[49] All medical courses now have places and entry pathways for Indigenous applicants and some are particularly focussed on this aspect.

The medical deans have since worked with Indigenous doctors to develop a specific curriculum framework about the health of Indigenous Australians which is now incorporated in the curricula of all Australian medical courses as a requirement of AMC accreditation.

The Australian Medical Association each year funds an Indigenous Peoples' Medical Scholarship valued at $10,000. Applicants must have completed at least their first year of medical studies.[50] For Indigenous students there are also the Puggy Hunter Memorial Scholarships valued at $15,000 per year.[51]

2.22 What does it cost to be a full fee paying domestic or international medical student?

Some Australian students have the resources to enrol in a full fee paying medical course, but this is only possible at private universities (University of Notre Dame and Bond University) and a limited number of the public medical courses (e.g. the University of Melbourne). The websites of individual medical schools should be consulted. The annual fees are set by each university: in 2019 Bond University quoted a total course fee over four and a half years of $391,144. At the University of Melbourne the four year course cost $285,184 based on 2019 figures while the four year course at Notre Dame University cost $143,952 and the four year course at Macquarie University will cost in the vicinity of $264,000. These fees do not cover the costs of accommodation, daily living and incidental expenses such as textbooks.

The cost of medical education for international medical students (IMS) who come to Australia must be borne by the students, unless they are supported by their country of origin. In general, the websites of each medical school that accepts IMS provide information about these costs. For example the annual cost of the University of Melbourne graduate entry 4 year degree in 2018 was $86,720.[52] In addition there are a number of websites (government sponsored and other) that provide this information.[53] The cost of living in Australia also needs to be considered as in 2019 this was estimated at $20,290 per year.

2.23 Coping with the psychology of going into debt and the reality of debt at graduation

The current system of funding of tertiary education in Australia means that most students graduate with a debt owed to the government that will be gradually repaid after commencing paid employment. The MABEL study (see Section 1.9) reported in 2010 that the average medical graduate educational debt was $27,710.[54] In 2019 it is likely to have risen to around $35,000–40,000. The experience of recent graduates is that this debt is usually easily managed and is repaid reasonably promptly. The amount to be repaid each year is determined as a percentage of annual income, starting at 1% for an income of $45,880 and rising to 5% for an annual income of over $70,000.[55]

Base salaries (to which will be added overtime and penalty rates) of new medical graduates (interns) vary across Australia, ranging in January 2019 from $67,950 in New South Wales to $78,479 in Western Australia.[56] Salaries are reviewed and updated regularly and it is thus likely that they will be higher when you graduate. HECS/HELP loans are also likely to be higher.

If you do not have generous family support, then it will be very important to take great care with your finances. Most medical students work part-time during some of or all the course. Finding suitable part-time work can be a challenge. A good starting point will be via the university student employment service. Employers who use this service usually have good insight into the lives of university students and may be more flexible and understanding of the pressures facing full time students. All medical courses are full-time so if possible you should try to minimise your hours of part-time work during semesters, especially Monday to Friday, so as not to jeopardise your training. Universities also provide advice about housing support, bursaries and loans. Many students find part-time work in the health fields (e.g. ward clerk, orderly, receptionist, phlebotomist), education (e.g. tutoring) or research and some may spend up to twenty hours per week doing so. Depending upon your financial situation, you may also be eligible for assistance from Centrelink via Youth Allowance (means tested and accessible until the age of 25) or Austudy (for students aged 25 years or more).[*]

Borrowing money from a bank can be considered but Australian banks will generally not lend money solely on the basis that you are likely to become a doctor; you will need another person with realisable assets to act as your guarantor. Your university will have an office where financial advice can be obtained and some universities provide low interest short term loans. For some students, this may be an option worthy of consideration, particularly for the more intensive clinical training years, as it will reduce your need to work part-time and make completing the course less onerous. A further option is to defer clinical studies for a year in order to work full time to save the money needed.

---

[*]   More information is available on the Centrelink website (www.centrelink.gov.au).

2.24 Are there any lateral entry pathways?

Some UG medical schools permit a small number of students each year to change career direction, within that university, and enter the medical course from another degree course. In addition, some UG medical schools accept applications from persons who have completed another undergraduate degree. For more detail, each university's website should be consulted. All GE medical courses require prior completion of an undergraduate degree.

2.25 My real wish is to be a medical researcher. Do I need a medical degree?

The simple answer to this question is 'No'. However, that answer needs to be qualified in relation to the nature of the research you have in mind. Broadly, there are two pathways to becoming a researcher in the field of medicine and medical sciences. Some medical graduates choose a career in full time medical research and forgo all or nearly all clinical work. Many of these, including some Australian medical graduates, have won Nobel prizes in medicine. In choosing such a path, these graduates will usually complete their training in a medical specialty (see Section 5.10) and then undertake a Doctor of Philosophy (PhD), learning to be a researcher under supervision. They then work alongside other scientists with PhDs who have not undertaken a medical degree.

The second pathway (not involving a medical degree) usually commences with an undergraduate science degree followed by an honour's year, possibly a Master's degree and then finally a PhD. The PhD experience of medical researchers in either pathway will be similar apart from the opportunity that the medical graduate PhD candidate has to choose a research theme that involves continuing direct contact with patients.

Some medical courses place considerable emphasis on the potential for their graduates to become successful medical researchers and virtually all GE courses now ensure that students engage in a 'hands on' research project over weeks or months. In addition, most UG medical courses offer an opportunity to spend an intercalated year in research and obtain an additional degree (e.g. a BMedSc). If you already envisage a career in academic medicine or a post at a teaching hospital after completion of specialist training, an intercalated year in research should be given consideration.

If you have an interest in medical research rather than an ambition to devote your career solely to medical research, you need to know that many medical graduates are able to combine part time clinical and/or laboratory research with active clinical practice. In preparation for the research element of their careers, doctors in training may opt to undertake a research degree such as a Master's degree or a PhD. While this career path is most often pursued by medical graduates employed full-time in university or hospital positions, it is not unknown for private medical practitioners to maintain an active role in research. In addition, clinical research by general practitioners into aspects of family practice is becoming a part of the lives of some general practitioners, usually through employment by, or affiliation with, a university academic department of general practice. Whatever path you choose to pursue an interest in research, you will be potentially making important contributions to improved health care. Without some doctors devoting their energies to research, health care will stagnate.

Attachment: The Australian medical schools

Care has been taken to accurately summarise the information contained on the websites of the medical schools listed below but you are strongly advised to examine each relevant website and make your own interpretation of the content. In addition, the provision of medical education is subject to continuous change: for example, the Federal Government has funded a network of rural clinical schools (linked to several existing medical schools) in the Murray-Darling Basin which should be opened by 2021.[57] These facilities will allow rural students to complete their entire course without having to relocate to an urban school.

Australian National University Medical School

https://programsandcourses.anu.edu.au/2019/program/8950XMCHD

The Australian National University in Canberra, ACT was established in 1946 but has only had a medical school since 2004. The medical course is graduate entry and is of four years duration. The number of commencing students in 2016 was 94 of whom 4 were international students. The school will accept up to twenty fee paying international students. The school does not accept full fee paying Australian students.

Other than an undergraduate degree, there are no prerequisites. Selection is based on a combination of weighted grade point average (GPA, a measure of academic performance during the undergraduate degree) and the score from GAMSAT as well as a semi-structured multi-station interview. The interview, which includes a group task, is rated as satisfactory or unsatisfactory. Bonus points are awarded for an honours year. Students wishing to be placed and supported in the rural stream (see below) are asked to provide a two-page autobiographical statement. An additional, separate interview is conducted for applicants to the rural clinical school. A separate admission process is in place for Indigenous applicants. Entry via the Bachelor of Health Science degree and the Bachelor of Philosophy degree is also available.

The course structure in years 1 and 2 is based on a combination of lectures and problem-based learning (PBL). Patient contact commences in year 1. In years 3 and 4, the teaching is described as case-based learning with clinical rotations. The University campus is in the Canberra suburb of Acton and the medical school is also located there. Clinical schools are located at Canberra Hospital and Calvary Hospital which is also in Canberra. There is a rural clinical school which uses facilities in Cooma, Goulburn, Bega, Young and the Eurobodalla. All students spend some time in a rural placement in year 3 but 25% of students (those who have been selected for the rural stream) spend all of year 3 at rural clinical school sites.

Bond University Medical School

https://bond.edu.au/program/medical-program

Bond University is Australia's first private university, established in 1989. Its campus is located at Robina on the Queensland Gold Coast. The medical school accepts both undergraduate and graduate entrants and the length of the course is a little less than five years. The course is composed of an initial Bachelor of Medical Studies (BMSt) degree of two years and eight months followed by a two-year Doctor of Medicine (MD) degree. The number of students commencing in 2016 was 101. Places in the BMSt/MD course are available only to domestic applicants but international students graduating in other health-related degrees may be accepted into the MD course. All students are full fee paying. The fees for year 2019 were $27,960 per semester, over 14 semesters (four years and eight months). Some assistance with fees is available and students can apply for some external scholarships.

Entry requirements include prerequisite subjects of chemistry, mathematics B (or equivalent) and English or a previous tertiary degree. Selection of undergraduates is based on the University Clinical Aptitude Test (UCAT)* score, academic performance and interview. Selection of graduate entrants is based on GPA from the previous degree and interview. Since 2018, selection is also based on psychometric testing, intended to assess emotional intelligence, and this testing is also used to select applicants for interview.

The course structure is problem-based learning (PBL) with early patient contact. The medical school is located on the Robina campus and clinical schools are located at the following hospitals: Gold Coast Hospital, Robina Hospital, Tweed Hospital, John Flynn Hospital, Allamanda Hospital, Pindara Hospital, and Wesley Hospital.

---

* UCAT is an admissions test used by the UCAT ANZ Consortium of universities in Australia and New Zealand for their medical, dental and clinical science degree programmes. For more information see Section 2.8.

Curtin University Medical School

https://study.curtin.edu.au/offering/course-ug-bachelor-of-medicine-bachelor-of-surgery--b-mbbsv1/

Curtin University is located in Western Australia with its main campus at Bentley, an inner suburb of Perth. Its medical school opened in 2018 as a five-year undergraduate entry course when 60 domestic students enrolled in first year. It is planned that first-year enrolments will increase by 10 students per year to a maximum of 110 in 2022. The medical school does not accept international students. Chemistry is a prerequisite subject and student selection is based on a combination of ATAR and UCAT scores and an interview. There are separate entry paths for Indigenous students and rural students and a mechanism for seeking equity for students from disadvantaged backgrounds.

The first year of the course is inter-professional taken with other health science students, but with separate units for each discipline and for medical students there is a unit on introduction to clinical practice. Second and third years cover the structure and function of the human body in health and disease, including transition into clinical settings. Fourth and final year are entirely clinical with placements at Midland Hospital, Royal Perth Hospital, Fiona Stanley Hospital, Peel Hospital, Fremantle Hospital, general practice clinics across the state, and rural medical settings.

Deakin University Medical School

https://www.deakin.edu.au/course/doctor-medicine

Deakin University is primarily located in Geelong in Victoria, with campuses also in Melbourne and Warrnambool. Its medical school, on the Geelong campus, is relatively young as the initial cohort of students commenced in 2008. The course is graduate entry and is of four years duration. There were 146 commencing students in 2016 of whom eight were international students.

Entry requirements include an undergraduate degree, a weighted GPA of at least 5 and a GAMSAT score of 50 in each section of the examination. Selection is based on a ranking of applicants according to a combination of weighted GPA, GAMSAT score and a multi station mini interview. Selection bonuses are awarded to applicants from a rural background, and those who have had previous clinical experience or have experienced financial disadvantage during their undergraduate degree. A minimum of 25% of places are set aside for students who qualify for the rural residency bonus. A separate entry path exists for Indigenous students.

The course structure is PBL-based with early patient contact. For years 1 and 2, students are based at the medical school on Deakin's Waurn Ponds campus in Geelong. Clinical schools are at Geelong University Hospital, Warrnambool Hospital, Ballarat Hospital, Box Hill Hospital (in Melbourne) and a rural community clinical school based at Warrnambool linked to rural general practices in Ararat, Horsham, Hamilton, Daylesford and Bacchus Marsh. The course overall has an emphasis on rural and regional medicine and aims to address the critical shortage of doctors in regional areas. A cohort of students spends all of year 3 at a rural general practice in Western Victoria. An elective term of 6 weeks is spent in year 4 and may be taken in Australia or overseas.

Flinders University Medical School
https://www.flinders.edu.au/study/courses/postgraduate-doctor-medicine/md-apply

Flinders University medical school home campus is situated in Bedford Park, Adelaide in South Australia. The medical course is co-located with Flinders Medical Centre. The medical course is of four years duration and the main admissions path is graduate entry (GE). However, school leavers can gain entry by first enrolling in a two-year Bachelor of Clinical Sciences degree and meeting satisfactory progress requirements. There is also a rural student entry pathway. Flinders University has an agreement with Charles Darwin University in Darwin that allows Northern Territory residents, especially Indigenous residents, to undertake the entire Flinders four-year degree in the Northern Territory. Some places in the NT program are bonded places sponsored by the Northern Territory government. In addition, Flinders is the only course that reserves places for students who hold humanitarian visas.

The number of students enrolled in first year in 2016 was 165 of whom 28 were international fee paying students. For either the Adelaide or Darwin programs, Indigenous applicants are encouraged to apply through an Indigenous Entry Stream (IES) that does not require GAMSAT. The entry requirement for the GE course is an undergraduate degree. Selection, other than via the IES, is based on a combination of weighted GPA, GAMSAT score and interview. Selection for high school-leavers into the six-year combined Bachelor of Clinical Sciences/Doctor of Medicine degree path is based on the Australian Tertiary Admissions Rank (or equivalent) and UCAT score.

The GE course structure includes two predominantly pre-clinical years with team-based learning followed by two years of clinical placements. There is emphasis on clinical skills and patient contact from year 1. Clinical schools are based at Flinders Medical Centre and in Mount Gambier, Renmark, Victor Harbour and Barossa (all in South Australia). In addition, Flinders Medical School conducts two clinical schools in the Northern Territory, one based at Royal Darwin Hospital, which provides community based medical education in urban Darwin and a second Northern Territory Rural Clinical School based at Alice Springs, Katherine and Gove. Among seven clinical rotations in fourth year, two elective terms may be taken either in Australia or overseas.

Griffith University Medical School
https://www.griffith.edu.au/study/health/medicine

Griffith University is located in Queensland and its health campus, the Centre for Medicine and Oral Health, is based in Southport on the Gold Coast, adjacent to the new Gold Coast University Hospital. The medical school, opened in 2005, is graduate entry and the course is of four years duration. The number of commencing students in 2016 was 176 of whom 19 were international students. The entry requirement is an undergraduate degree GPA above 5. Selection is based on a combination of GAMSAT score and a multi-station interview. The medical course also has a separate entry path for Indigenous students, priority access for rural students and offers a combined MD/PhD path for selected students. From 2019, the medical course may also be undertaken at the Sunshine Coast University Hospital and Sunshine Coast Health Institute.

The course structure includes two preclinical years with PBL and two clinical years. Early patient contact commences in year 1 with hospital-based training as well as community based training. Clinical placements are based at the following hospitals: Gold Coast University Hospital, Sunshine Coast University Hospital, Logan Hospital, Tweed Hospital, and QEII Hospital as well as rural hospitals at Warwick, Gympie, Kingaroy, Stanthorpe, Dalby and Beaudesert. Elective terms are two five weeks rotations in fourth year and these can be local, rural or international. Selective terms are two four-week rotations based locally.

James Cook University Medical School

https://www.jcu.edu.au/courses-and-study/courses/bachelor-of-medicine,-bachelor-of-surgery

James Cook University has two major campuses in Townsville and Cairns, as well as smaller campuses and study centres in other locations in Queensland and overseas. The MBBS is an undergraduate course of six years' duration and is split between several locations. The course focuses on rural and remote health, Indigenous health and tropical medicine. The number of commencing students in 2016 was 209 of whom 38 were international students.

The first three years are based in Townsville, year 4 is based in Townsville and Cairns, and years 5 and 6 are based in clinical schools in Townsville,

Cairns, Mackay or Darwin as well as extended placements in small rural and remote communities. This medical school does not participate in the UCAT consortium and applications must be made directly to the university by September 30 of the year before commencement.

Prerequisite subjects are English, mathematics B and chemistry while the study of physics and biology is described as highly desirable Student selection is through a combination of a written application, interview and academic results. There is a separate selection pathway for Aboriginal and Torres Strait Islander students.

While the course broadly comprises three pre-clinical years and three clinical years, patient contact begins in year 1 and clinical attachments, including rural and remote placements, are undertaken in every year of the course.

Macquarie University Medical School

https://courses.mq.edu.au/2019/domestic/postgraduate/doctor-of-medicine

Macquarie University is located in the Sydney suburb of North Ryde. The medical course is a four-year graduate entry degree. The medical school is new and the first students were enrolled in 2018. It is anticipated that the maximum enrolment each first year will be limited to 60 students (40 domestic and 20 international). The medical course is full fee paying for both domestic and international students. The medical school is part of the GAMSAT consortium and uses GEMSAS as its entry point. However, applicants have to have completed prerequisite courses in human anatomy and human physiology. Selection is then based on GPA, GAMSAT score and multiple mini interview. There are score adjustments for Indigenous and rural applicants and a separate entry path for Indigenous students.

The primary location of the medical school is a university hospital on the campus known as Macquarie Health described as 'Australia's first university-led, integrated health campus, where learning is fully integrated with outstanding patient-centred clinical care, and active health and medical research'. Clinical rotations are also provided through the Royal North Shore Hospital, the Northern Sydney Local Health District and the Apollo Hospital in Hyderabad, India.

Monash University Medical School

http://www.med.monash.edu.au/

Monash University's main campus is in the south-eastern Melbourne suburb of Clayton in Victoria. The faculty conducts school-leaver (undergraduate) entry programs at the Clayton and Malaysian* campuses and a graduate entry program, the first year of which is based at Churchill in West Gippsland. After completing the first year at Churchill, the graduate entrants join the undergraduate entrants in the third year of their course. The undergraduate courses are of 5 years duration and the graduate entry course is 4 years. In 2016, there were 304 commencing students in the undergraduate entry course at Clayton of whom 62 were international students while in the postgraduate entry course there were 86 commencing students of whom 11 were international students.

Prerequisite subjects for the undergraduate course are English and chemistry. Selection for this course is based on the UCAT score for domestic students, the ISAT[†] score for international applicants, academic performance and multi mini interview. A bridging course in biology is provided for students who have not studied this at high school.

The graduate entry course is available to students who have completed a Monash degree in biomedical science, pharmacy, physiotherapy or science (with specified units completed) and to international students. Selection for the graduate entry course is based on GPA, GAMSAT score for domestic applicants (GAMSAT or MCAT[‡] score for international applicants) and

---

* Australian residents are not eligible to enrol in the Monash Malaysian program.

† ISAT refers to the International Students Admission Test. It is a computer-based test conducted by ACER to assist Australian universities in assessing the capacity of applicants for academic success.

‡ MCAT refers to the USA Medical Colleges Admission Test which is the equivalent of GAMSAT.

multi mini interview. Some places are allocated to Indigenous students, students from rural areas and disadvantaged students.

All courses are integrated, with basic sciences being taught in the early years and clinical rotations in later years. Patient contact begins in Year 1. Clinical schools exist at a large number of locations in urban Melbourne (e.g. at the Alfred Hospital, Monash Medical Centre and Box Hill Hospital) and rural Victoria (e.g. Bendigo Base Hospital, Mildura Base Hospital, Latrobe Regional Hospital at Traralgon). All students are exposed to rural medicine and a cohort of students is given the opportunity to spend up to two years at a rural site. An elective term of six weeks duration takes place in final year.

University of Adelaide Medical School
https://www.adelaide.edu.au/degree-finder/bmbbs_bmbbs.html

The University of Adelaide, South Australia, is centrally located in North Terrace, Adelaide and the medical school is nearby. The medical course is undergraduate entry and is of six years duration. In 2016 the number of commencing students was 160 of whom 31 were international students.

Prerequisite subjects include biology or chemistry or mathematics. The entry requirement is an ATAR greater than 90 (or equivalent). Students are selected based on a combination of UCAT score, ATAR and interview. Places are reserved for rural students and graduates from the university's Bachelor of Health and Medical Sciences course. There is a separate entry pathway for Indigenous students.

Clinical skills training in third year is conducted primarily in the public teaching hospitals, followed by a variety of clinical placements in years 4–6 (some compulsory, some elective). Clinical schools are located at Royal Adelaide Hospital, Queen Elizabeth Hospital, Lyell McEwen Hospital and Modbury Hospital (all in or near to Adelaide) and in Whyalla. Some students will be able to undertake year 5 in a rural setting. Year 6 is focused on what students need to know for their internship. The major exam is conducted at the end of year 5, and with the pressure of exams reduced, final year students can focus on their clinical practice and professional development.

University of Melbourne Medical School

http://www.medicine.unimelb.edu.au/

The University of Melbourne has the oldest medical school in Australia having been established in 1862. Its medical course has recently changed to a graduate entry course. At the same time, the University decided that graduates would be awarded the MD (Doctor of Medicine) in place of the previous MBBS.* The course duration is four years, preceded by a three year Bachelor of Biomedicine degree covering the subjects of anatomy, physiology and biochemistry. The medical school is on the university campus which is located in Carlton very close to the central business district. In 2016, 353 students commenced the first year of the graduate degree of whom 44 were international students.

Student selection is based on a combination of GAMSAT score, GPA and multi mini interview. While the Bachelor of Biomedicine is the most obvious pathway to entry, graduates with other degrees have been successful applicants. However all those accepted must meet the prerequisite of having completed an undergraduate degree with studies in anatomy, physiology and biochemistry at second-year level (or equivalent).

The course structure includes a year of case-based integrated bioscience and clinical learning held on the university campus followed by three clinical years. The medical school has clinical schools at the

---

* At that point in time, all other graduate entry medical course qualifications were deemed to be second undergraduate degrees. The University of Melbourne MD qualification was set at the Master's level under the Australian Qualifications Framework (https://www.aqf.edu.au/) necessitating a considerable research component in the course. The MD was thus deemed to be a postgraduate degree and for this reason the university was permitted to offer the course to full fee-paying domestic students. The Australian Qualifications Framework requirements are distinct from the accreditation requirements of the Australian Medical Council; the latter focus on the capacity of the medical course to prepare graduates for the intern year.

following Melbourne hospitals: (a) Royal Melbourne Hospital, St Vincent's Hospital, Austin Hospital and Epworth Hospital forming the Inner East Zone; (b) Western Hospital, Sunshine Hospital and Northern Hospital forming the Western Zone; and (c) a Rural Zone with a clinical school for which the Goulburn Valley Hospital at Shepparton, the Wangaratta Hospital, Ballarat Hospital and Bendigo Hospital form the basis. A cohort of students participate in an extended rural exposure in third year with placements including Shepparton, Murchison, Echuca, Wangaratta, Mt Beauty, Cobram, Corowa, Yarrawonga, Benalla or Mansfield. Students may also spend time at the Royal Women's Hospital, Royal Children's Hospital and Mercy Hospital for Women. In the first half of the final year students must undertake full-time research.

University of New South Wales Medical School

http://med.unsw.edu.au/

The University of New South Wales is located in the southern Sydney suburb of Kensington and the medical school is located there. The medical course is predominantly undergraduate entry and is of six years duration, with students completing a combined Bachelor of Medical Studies and Doctor of Medicine. There is a second graduate entry path for up to 10 students who first enrol in the Bachelor of Medical Science (BMedSc) degree. These students, who will be selected based on a combination of their grades in the first two years of BMedSc, their UCAT score and interview, will enter year 4 of the medical course. In 2016, there were 270 commencing students in the undergraduate course of whom 84 were international students.

There are no formal prerequisite year 12 subjects but chemistry is recommended. Student selection for the undergraduate course is based on a combination of year 12 achievement, UCAT score and an interview. Places are reserved for rural students and there is a separate pathway for Indigenous applicants. Successful Indigenous applicants must take a three-week residential pre-medicine program.

The undergraduate course is highly integrated based on scenario groups, clinical groups, lectures and practical classes. There is early patient contact from year 1. The medical school has clinical schools at Prince of Wales Hospital in Randwick, St Vincent's Hospital, Darlinghurst, St George Hospital, Kogarah, Sutherland Hospital Caringbah, Sydney Children's Hospital in Randwick, the Royal Hospital for Women in Randwick, Liverpool Hospital, Liverpool, Fairfield Hospital, Fairfield and Bankstown Hospital, Bankstown. In addition a number of regional and rural hospitals in NSW are used for clinical teaching in Wagga Wagga, Port Macquarie Base Hospital, Coffs Harbour Hospital and Griffith. Students now have the option of completing all years of the course at the Port Macquarie campus.

University of Newcastle and University of New England Joint Medical Program

www.newcastle.edu.au/jmp and www.une.edu.au/jmp

These two universities in the state of New South Wales offer the Joint Medical Program (JMP) as an undergraduate entry course of five years duration, leading to the Bachelor of Medical Sciences and Doctor of Medicine degree. Students are based at either the University of Newcastle main campus at Callaghan in Newcastle or at the University of New England in Armidale. In 2016, there were 211 students commencing first year, of whom 26 were international students.

There are no prerequisite subjects. Selection of academically qualified applicants (i.e. qualified via their ATAR score or university grade average) for admission to the program is based on performance in the UCAT following which applicants will be selected for a personal qualities assessment at one or other university campus. On the day of assessment, applicants must complete an online personal qualities assessment[58] followed by an eight station multiple skills assessment. The JMP actively seeks applications from students with a rural or remote background and reserves places each year for Indigenous students.

The course structure integrates basic sciences with clinical medicine and is PBL-based with early patient contact starting in Semester 1. There are six clinical schools where placement can be undertaken: three rural clinical schools in Armidale, Tamworth and Taree, and three urban clinical schools in Maitland, Hunter Clinical School (Newcastle) and the Central Coast Clinical School.

University of Notre Dame Australia, Fremantle Medical School

https://www.notredame.edu.au/programs/fremantle/school-of-medicine/postgraduate/doctor-of-medicine

The University of Notre Dame is located in Fremantle, south of Perth, in Western Australia. The medical school is also located primarily in Fremantle. The medical course is graduate entry and of four years duration. In 2016, there were 110 commencing domestic students. The school does not accept international students at present.

The entry prerequisite is an undergraduate degree with a GPA of at least 5.2. Student selection is based on a combination of personal qualities and motivation (applicants must provide a portfolio), weighted GPA, GAMSAT score and a multi mini-interview. The medical school has a philosophy of seeking to graduate doctors prepared to work in underserviced areas and Indigenous and rural students are encouraged to apply.

The course structure involves two preclinical years with PBL followed by two clinical years.

Affiliated urban hospitals include Fiona Stanley Hospital, St John of God Hospital in Subiaco, St John of God Hospital, Murdoch, St John of God Hospital, Midland, Armadale Hospital, Hollywood Private Hospital and Royal Perth Hospital. Rural clinical schools are located at Kalgoorlie, Port Hedland, Busselton, Broome, Derby, Bunbury, Geraldton, Albany, Narrogin, Northam, Carnavon, Esperance, Kununurra and Karratha.

University of Notre Dame Australia, Sydney Medical School

https://www.notredame.edu.au/about/schools/sydney/medicine

The University of Notre Dame has a second medical school in Sydney, NSW. The medical school buildings are in Darlinghurst, Sydney. The course is graduate entry and is of four years duration. In 2016, there were 118 domestic students who commenced the course. Applications from international students were accepted from 2019.

The entry prerequisite is an undergraduate degree and selection is based on a portfolio regarding personal qualities and motivation combined with GPA, GAMSAT score and a multi mini-interview. There is a separate pathway for applications from Indigenous students.

The course structure is PBL-based, supported by lectures and clinical skills sessions. There is early patient contact. All students undertake a supervised applied medical research project during the course. The medical school has several urban and rural clinical schools. The urban schools include the St Vincent's & Mater Clinical School at St Vincent's Hospital, the Auburn Clinical School located at Auburn Hospital and the Hawkesbury Clinical School located at Hawkesbury Health Service, all in NSW, and the Melbourne Clinical School at Werribee Mercy Hospital in Victoria. The rural clinical schools include the Lithgow Clinical School at Lithgow Hospital and the Wagga Wagga Clinical School at Calvary Health Care Riverina, both in NSW, and the Ballarat Clinical School at St John of God Hospital, Ballarat in Victoria.

University of Queensland Medical School

https://future-students.uq.edu.au/study/program/Doctor-of-Medicine-5578?year=2019

The University of Queensland is situated at St Lucia in Brisbane with additional campuses at Ipswich, Gatton and Herston. The medical school is at Herston adjacent to a hospital complex that includes the Royal Brisbane and Women's Hospital. The medical course is graduate entry and of four years duration. In 2016, there were 404 commencing students of whom 83 were international students. In addition to graduate entry, there is also a provisional entry pathway for school leavers.

For graduate entry the prerequisite is a previous degree. Selection of students is based primarily on the GAMSAT score with GPA being used to separate students with the same GAMSAT score. As at 2019, there are no interviews but a multi mini-interview is soon to be introduced as are prerequisite subjects. In addition the medical school provides targeted access for Aboriginal and Torres Strait Islanders and students from rural and northern Australia.

Provisional entry to the graduate course is available based on secondary school achievement and UCAT score but successful applicants must complete their first degree at the University of Queensland in the minimum time and with a GPA of 5.00 to be admitted to the medical course.

The clinical years of the course may involve placements at a wide range of institutions in Brisbane, other towns and rural Queensland. These include the Royal Brisbane and Women's Hospital, Lady Cilento Children's Hospital, Greenslopes Private Hospital, Mater Hospital, Ipswich Hospital, Prince Charles Hospital, Redcliffe Hospital, Caboolture Hospital, Holy Spirit Northside Hospital, Princess Alexandra Hospital, Queen Elizabeth II Hospital, Redland Hospital, Sunshine Coast University Hospital, Wesley Hospital, St Andrew's War Memorial Hospital and 200 general practices throughout central and south-east Queensland. In addition there is a rural clinical school with bases in Bundaberg, Hervey Bay, Rockhampton and Toowoomba. Students may also have the option of placement at UQ Ochsner Clinical School located in Louisiana, USA.

University of Sydney Medical School

https://sydney.edu.au/courses/courses/pc/doctor-of-medicine.html

The University of Sydney is situated in Camperdown close to the central business district and is the oldest university in Australia. The medical course is graduate entry and is of four years duration. In 2016, there were 339 commencing students of whom 92 were international students. In 2020 a new MD curriculum and course structure will be introduced. The program will maintain the best aspects of the current course, while enhancing learning opportunities through earlier clinical exposure, new research opportunities, and immersive clinical placements in the last year of the program, preparing students for practice as a doctor.

The entry requirement is an undergraduate degree with a GPA of 5.5 or above. Student selection is based on a combination of GAMSAT score and assessment by multiple mini interview. There is targeted access for Indigenous and rural applicants. Applicants must apply directly to the University and be interviewed by the University to be considered for a place. As a biomedical science degree is not a prerequisite, a foundation course is available to all students on enrolment to assure adequate knowledge in anatomy, physiology and molecular and cellular biology.

A limited number of places are held for school leavers under the Combined Medicine option. These places may be taken up after satisfactory completion of the Bachelor of Science (Advanced), Bachelor of Medical Science, Bachelor of Arts (Advanced) (Honours) or the Bachelor of Music Studies degree at the University of Sydney. The admission criteria for this path involve performance in ATAR (or equivalent) and performance at interview. To be considered, you must have a very high ATAR or equivalent.

The course structure is PBL-based with early patient contact. The medical school is based in Camperdown with urban clinical schools at Royal Prince Alfred Hospital and adjacent hospitals, Concord Repatriation General Hospital, Westmead Hospital, the Children's Hospital at Westmead, Nepean Hospital, Royal North Shore Hospital and Sydney Adventist Hospital, and a rural clinical school with campuses at Broken Hill, Dubbo, Lismore, Orange and Bathurst.

University of Tasmania Medical School

https://www.utas.edu.au/courses/chm/courses/m3n-bachelor-of-medicine-and-bachelor-of-surgery

The University of Tasmania is located at Sandy Bay in Hobart as is the medical school. The medical course is undergraduate entry and is of five years duration. In 2016 the school enrolled 124 first year students, of whom 21 were international students.

Prerequisites include year 12 chemistry and English (including communications, literature and writing). Student selection is based on a combination of UCAT score and academic achievement (a minimum ATAR score of 95 or higher). Tertiary entry is available to students who undertake the University of Tasmania Bachelor of Medical Research degree. There are separate application paths for Indigenous students and rural students.

Course structure is based on the first three years being spent at the university and the last two spent in hospitals. The medical school has clinical schools at the Royal Hobart Hospital and in Launceston, and a rural clinical school in the north-west of Tasmania.

University of Western Australia Medical School

https://study.uwa.edu.au/courses/doctor-of-medicine

The University of Western Australia is located at Crawley in Perth and the medical school is based at the adjacent Queen Elizabeth 11 Medical Centre. The medical course is a four-year graduate entry program. In 2016, there were 237 commencing students of whom 25 were international students.

For entry, an undergraduate degree with a GPA of at least 5.5 is required. It is recommended that students have basic knowledge of physics, chemistry and biology. Selection is based on academic performance, GAMSAT score and a structured interview. There is a separate pathway for school leavers with an ATAR of 99 or equivalent and a separate pathway for rural students, both involving applicants to sit the UCAT.

Successful applicants for these pathways will have a place on the Doctor of Medicine course on the condition they complete a UWA Bachelor's degree with a GPA of at least 5.5. There is also an alternative entry pathway for Indigenous applicants, providing a bridging course and not involving UCAT or GAMSAT.

The course structure is described as an integrated curriculum with early patient contact. Clinical schools beyond the Queen Elizabeth II Medical Centre are based at Albany, Broome, Bunbury, Derby, Esperance, Geraldton, Kalgoorlie, Karratha, Narrogin and Port Hedland. In year 3, a quarter of the students are allocated to rural hospitals and general practices.

Western Sydney University Medical School

https://www.westernsydney.edu.au/future/study/how-to-apply/md-applicants.html

Western Sydney University has six campuses across greater western Sydney and the medical school is located on the Campbelltown campus. The medical course is undergraduate entry and is of five years duration. It now leads to a double degree – Bachelor of Clinical Science and Doctor of Medicine. In 2016, there were 133 commencing students of whom 24 were international students. There are no prerequisite subjects although chemistry is recommended. Selection of students is based on a combination of academic achievement, UCAT score and a multi-station mini interview. Applicants from Greater Western Sydney region are favoured and Indigenous applicants are encouraged to apply. Five places are available to Indigenous students.

The course structure includes half a day per week in hospitals in the first two preclinical years and full-time clinical exposure in years 3 to 5. Clinical schools are based at Campbelltown Hospital, Blacktown Hospital and Mt Druitt Hospital and there are rural clinical schools at Bathurst and Lismore for years 4/5 study. Affiliated hospitals include Camden Hospital, Fairfield Hospital, Liverpool Hospital and Bankstown/Lidcombe Hospital.

Students generally spend the most time at Campbelltown and Blacktown Hospitals. Some students may be allocated to rural placements based at Lismore or Bathurst for 12 months during their last two years.

University of Wollongong Medical School

https://smah.uow.edu.au/medicine/future/md/UOW027247.html

Wollongong is located south of Sydney in New South Wales. The medical school is located on the Wollongong campus with an additional campus at Shoalhaven. The medical course is graduate entry and is of four years duration. In 2016, there were 88 commencing students of whom 13 were international students.

The only entry requirement is an undergraduate degree with a GPA of 5 or above. Student selection is based on a combination of weighted GPA, GAMSAT score, a portfolio and a structured interview. Ranking for interview is also influenced by the score in an online test CASPer[59] designed to assess personal and professional traits, such as ethics, empathy and communication.

Students who can demonstrate a link to rural, remote or regional areas are favoured and there is targeted access for Indigenous students.

The course structure is described as case-based learning, supplemented with lectures, small group learning, clinical skills classes, anatomy laboratories and clinical placements. Clinical schools are based at the Wollongong Hospital, Shoalhaven District Hospital, Bulli Hospital, Shellharbour Hospital, Port Kembla Hospital and Bowral Hospital as well as in general practices and community health centres in the region.

THE STRUCTURE AND CONTENT OF THE MEDICAL COURSE

In this section I provide a broad outline of what you will be learning during your course, describe the various educational methods you will become familiar with, and depict the process by which a novice student gradually becomes a medical practitioner, one entitled to be registered with the Medical Board of Australia. The section also discusses the expectations placed on medical students and provides practical advice for students with families and students with a disability.

3.1 The ethical and professional standards expected of medical students

In commencing the study of medicine and especially when contact with patients begins, you need to be aware that you are on the path to joining a profession that has high ethical and professional standards. Your studies will cover the standards expected of doctors. Importantly most of those standards also apply to medical students. In addition, the AMSA has developed a code of ethics for medical students first published in 2003.[1]

The AMSA code outlines eight principles of conduct:

Medical students should:

- respect the needs, values and culture of patients they encounter during their training
- never exploit patients or their families
- hold clinical information in confidence
- obtain informed consent from patients before involving them in any aspect of training
- appreciate the limits of their role in the clinical setting and in the community
- respect the staff who teach and assist them in their clinical training
- adhere to the ethical principles in the appropriate national and international guidelines, if involved in clinical research
- maintain their personal integrity and well-being.

The full code has detailed explanations about how these principles are to be applied in practice.

Some Australian medical schools ask their students to read and sign a detailed code of student conduct; for example, James Cook University.[2] There are a number of other ethical guidelines written for doctors that are also relevant to medical students. Their relevance increases as the medical course evolves, and as students interact more closely with patients and other health professionals while learning of the professional behaviours expected of doctors. Included in these are guidelines on relationships between drug companies and doctors. *Good Medical Practice: A Code of Conduct for Doctors in Australia*[3] mentioned already in Section 1 states 'Good medical practice involves recognising that pharmaceutical and other medical marketing influences doctors and being aware of ways in which your practice may be being influenced'. You will undoubtedly be exposed as a student to 'educational' overtures from the pharmaceutical industry[4] and you are likely to be dismayed by how willingly doctors convince themselves that they are immune to such overtures, when the evidence to the contrary is powerful.

More detailed information about the ethical and legal obligations of medical students can be found in Chapter 4 of an Australian textbook entitled *Good Medical Practice: Professionalism, Ethics and Law.*[5]

Section 3.10 below discusses medical student misconduct and the approach taken by the medical schools to allegations of misconduct.

3.2 What subjects will I be studying, how will I learn and how will I be assessed?

The subjects that you will need to learn about are most readily identified in the curricula of traditional undergraduate medical courses and have usually been divided into pre-clinical (basic sciences) and clinical phases. Subjects covered in the pre-clinical phase include anatomy, physiology, biochemistry, histology, immunology, molecular biology, microbiology, pharmacology and pathology. You will also study epidemiology, statistics, psychology and sociology. In the clinical phase, you will be learning about how to interview, examine and communicate with patients and how to diagnose and treat a range of common conditions in settings including internal medicine, surgery, paediatrics, psychiatry, obstetrics and gynaecology and general practice. You will also be instructed in and expected to develop appropriate attitudes to, and understanding of, professional, ethical and legal issues in medical practice. The individual pre-clinical subjects identified above may be less readily visible in the integrated problem-based learning methods used in many of the medical courses (see below).

The range of basic science subjects that underpin much of modern medical practice means that graduate entry medical students whose first degree did not cover this material in any depth have to work harder in the early years of the course to keep up or catch up. Some graduate entry medical schools offer bridging courses to assist those students.

In the early phase of clinical training, you are likely to feel overwhelmed by the total amount of material you will need to learn. These feelings are common to all students and will gradually recede as you gain more experience and as you begin to appreciate that by using general principles already learned, many seemingly difficult problems can be solved. In addition, you should remember that the aim of your medical course is to prepare you for internship and not for independent medical practice. Learning continues in the intern and early postgraduate years, and indeed for the rest of your career.

Some of the teaching you will encounter will be familiar to you, e.g. class room lectures, tutorials and demonstrations, while other methods of learning may not be. Teaching and learning methods include problem-based learning (see below), team-based learning, self-directed learning, clinical skills laboratories, teaching with the patient present, simulation and role play. The last two approaches are methods of learning about patient-doctor communication and interaction using actors, fellow students or computer modulated simulators. Students rate clinically based teaching very highly.[6]

As will be discussed again later, one of the aspects of clinical medicine that new doctors find disturbing is that there is often much uncertainty in making a diagnosis, offering treatments and answering questions about prognosis. Unless this is well-addressed in the medical course, it can be disconcerting and stressful to medical students and new doctors alike to find that despite what is sometimes depicted as the precise application of scientific methods, the 'real world' of clinical medicine is very different.[7]

One facet of clinical training that some students avoid or ignore is the opportunity to talk to and, with their permission, examine as many patients as possible. Most patients, especially those in hospital, are willing to give time to student doctors as they are aware that this helps to train the nation's future doctors. This is valuable experience as it will increase your confidence in your communication skills, improve your ability to examine patients, and broaden your exposure to all the illnesses that befall people. Most students who grasp this opportunity find it easier and more rewarding to pair up with a like-minded student.

Assessment methods vary among the medical schools but usually include written assignments such as essays, short answer questions and multiple choice questions; clinical assessments such as 'long' and 'short' cases* and objective structured clinical examinations (OSCE);† reports of tutors and other observers; and assessment of cases seen or skills mastered via methods such as portfolios‡ and logbooks.§

3.3 What is problem-based learning?

Problem-based learning (PBL) is a learning approach pioneered in the medical course at McMaster University in Canada and has since become widely used in medical courses around the world.[8] It is now used as one of several methods of learning in many Australian medical courses.[9] It has several distinctive features including: the need for students to work collaboratively in groups, preferably small; problems are explored in depth over a period of a week or two; and the role of tutors as group facilitators and not content experts, supporting the group in self-directed learning. This learning is usually initiated by a clinical case (the 'problem') and the student group is then expected to explore the clinical aspects of the case as well as master the basic science knowledge needed to understand the case. For example, a week might be devoted to a case of a child with severe meningitis and, in exploring the case, you will be expected to not only learn about diagnosis and treatment but also about the relevant microbiology, anatomy, pathophysiology, pharmacology and epidemiology. Such a case

---

*   A 'long' case refers to the student being asked to take a detailed history from and conduct a full physical examination of a patient and then present the findings to an examiner. A 'short' case refers to a similar assessment but the student is confined to taking a brief history or completing a physical examination confined to one body system such as the respiratory system.

†   In an OSCE, students progress through a circuit of 'stations' where each station assesses a different clinical skill (e.g. communication, physical examination, interpretation of investigations etc.) and the examiner at each station uses predetermined criteria to award a mark.

‡   A portfolio is a personal record of a student that could include accounts of clinical experiences and reflections on what the student is seeing and learning or having difficulty learning (Snadden D and Thomas M. The use of portfolio learning in medical education. *Medical Teacher*, 1998, 20: 192–9.).

§   A logbook refers to the systematic recording of procedures observed or procedures performed under supervision.

might also be used to explore issues such as communicating bad news to parents, the legal rights of minors, and other themes. Given the potential scope of fields of knowledge that may need to be explored, it should not surprise that students new to this method of learning find this aspect disconcerting.

As an approach to learning, it is heavily dependent upon the medical school having sufficient resources to support PBL and on having facilitators /tutors who are trained and committed to the role expected of them. As a learning approach it has its enthusiastic adherents and its critics. In addition, there is confusion about the precise definition of PBL.[10] Some research has been done on its effectiveness but given the number of variables affecting medical training, the benefits are difficult to evaluate. A 2008 review of published research concluded that PBL has positive benefits on doctor competence, predominantly in the areas of coping with uncertainty, appreciation of legal and ethical issues, communication skills and continuing self-directed learning.[11] This review noted that new medical graduates have been reported to assess themselves as having less content knowledge of medicine when compared to peers who attended non-PBL courses.

A study of students in two UK medical schools, one of which used PBL and the other did not, reported that students found some aspects of PBL courses stressful, such as not knowing what was expected of them and being involved in student groups lacking adequate facilitation. On the other hand these students were less likely to feel a lack of encouragement from teachers and less likely to report that the course fostered a sense of anonymity or isolation.[12]

In Australia, the AME Study reported that some senior doctors felt that PBL courses contributed to new graduates being less well prepared in basic sciences such as anatomy and physiology. In the same study, junior doctors who had graduated from PBL courses felt better prepared for the psychosocial issues encountered in practice, whereas their peers who had graduated from courses with traditional teaching methods felt more knowledgeable about basic sciences.[13]

Over time PBL has evolved and its use in medical courses has become less rigid and less extensive. In some courses it is now partially supplanted by other approaches including team-based learning and case-based learning. The emphasis is still on group learning, facilitated by a teacher with relevant expertise.[14]

3.4 Who will be our lecturers and teachers?

A wide range of people will be your teachers, lecturers, instructors, supervisors and tutors. In your clinical rotations, most of these people will be doctors. There is a long tradition in medicine, dating back to the time of Hippocrates, of doctors teaching medical students and teaching remains an obligation identified in the code of ethics of the Australian Medical Association.[15] The code reads in part 'Honour your obligation to pass on your professional knowledge and skills to colleagues and students'. Although most doctors willingly accept a teaching load, they are paid at relatively low rates or not at all for their teaching. Most have not had any formal training as educators and not all are effective teachers. The majority of your teachers will be good role models but a minority may be less than ideal and the behaviour of some towards you or to patients may cause you distress. Coping with such stress and distress is discussed in Section 4.

As a medical student and especially as an intern (see Section 5), you will also have the opportunity to work closely with and learn from registrars* and other junior doctors who graduated ahead of you (see Section 5.8 for a more detailed description of the terminology used to categorise junior doctors). Registrars are generally in the hospital full time and play a very important role in teaching and role modelling as well as in patient care. Most are excellent and enthusiastic teachers and mentors. You may well find that some of them have a greater influence on the direction of your career than the more senior doctors you will meet. As interns you may

---

* The title registrar refers to doctors in training programs beyond the second or third postgraduate year. Most trainees hold the title of registrar for 3–6 years and during this time will be given increasing independence and responsibility.

unfortunately encounter registrars who are less than helpful and even a few who engage in bullying or other unacceptable forms of professional conduct. Some may be so involved in studying for their post-graduate examinations that you will feel unsupported.

You will get more out of this wide variety of teaching and instruction if you remember that at university the responsibility for learning is yours and not the teacher's. Busy clinicians involved in your teaching are more likely to respond if you show enthusiasm and interest. In contact with these clinicians you should consciously think about the role modelling that you encounter and what behaviours you should try to emulate, or not emulate, in the case of poor role models.

3.5 What else can I expect during my course? Are there other aspects I should be aware of?

For students entering a medical course directly from school, the experience of learning at university and the independence of the life of the university student can result in difficulties and distractions. These can lead previously highly achieving students to fail one or more subjects and the need to repeat a year. However, it is much more difficult to get into medical school than it is to pass the course. Failure rates are low and you should be optimistic about how you will progress. In general universities do not provide 'teaching' as experienced in high school but instead provide students with the materials and opportunities for self-directed learning. This can lead to you feeling disoriented and/or anxious in that the curriculum is not always precisely spelled out. Unlike school, there are no teachers supervising attendance or closely monitoring your progress, so the new freedom can lead to you being distracted and not completing enough work to progress to the next year. Some tips on methods of study, including joining a study group, can be found in Section 4.9. Taking an active part in the life of the university (for example by joining the medical students' society or a sporting club or a political group) is important for your personal development but these activities will need to be kept in balance with the need to study.

Much of medical students' learning takes place away from the university campus at hospitals and other clinical sites, especially in the later years of the course, when the curriculum takes you into daily contact with patients. Seeing very sick patients, and even before if you study anatomy with cadavers, you may experience a gradual change of emotional response to what you see and experience; some writers describe this as a form of de-humanisation, distancing or emotional detachment, developing in response to a need to manage overwhelming emotions. This change, which may be even more marked in the early years after graduation, may not be noticed by you but can be perceived by patients as representing disinterest in them as people and lack of care and empathy. Equally important for the caring and empathic doctor is the opposite response where the doctor can become emotionally over-involved in the care of patients. This can have negative consequences by making patients too dependent, clouding the doctor's clinical judgement, and even the over-stepping of boundaries by developing a personal rather than a professional relationship with a patient.

For a number of reasons, much medical student contact with patients still takes place in hospitals, even though in their future careers the majority of doctors will practise medicine away from the hospital environment either fully or most of the time. This narrow experience of the practice of medicine can lead to medical students being unaware of and perhaps having negative attitudes to all the interesting and rewarding work of general medical practice. Unfortunately, these negative attitudes can be reinforced by some hospital specialists who have a poor understanding of the importance of general practice in the Australian health care system and of the challenges faced by general practitioners.

Because doctors are held in high esteem by the community, as a medical student you might find yourself at times being regarded as a 'special' person following a special calling, for example by friends and relatives and even thinking this yourself. This feeling can be reinforced if nearly all of your time is spent with peers and as a result, friendships and relationships that keep you grounded in the real world are neglected.

As a medical student, you might be approached by friends and family for 'medical advice', thus reinforcing this feeling of specialness. You should avoid attempting to give any specific advice in such situations, although you may be in a position to urge people to seek proper medical attention. Most medical schools encourage or insist that early in the course, students obtain a certificate in first aid and this should be the limit of clinical care to be offered (outside the learning environment) until the point of medical registration.

It is not unusual for medical students when learning about clinical medicine to begin to imagine that they are suffering from the very disease they have been learning about, worrying for example that they may have a mental health disorder or a cancer such as leukaemia that can afflict younger patients. This is sufficiently common to be known informally as the 'medical student syndrome'.[16] Knowing that this can happen to you may help reduce the chance of it happening. However, persistent symptoms should not be ignored and independent medical advice should be sought, preferably from your own general practitioner.

Unfortunately a minority of clinical teachers and supervisors of medical students and young doctors exhibit conduct with patients which may distress students. This can include poor communication and rudeness and abruptness with patients, failing to obtain the consent of the patient to be seen and examined by students, and lack of awareness of patient discomfort. Some of these negative role models may occupy positions of high authority, and may also be admired for other attributes such as technical or procedural skills, leaving you confused as to what is and is not acceptable professional behaviour.

In addition some clinical teachers engage in bullying behaviour towards junior doctors, nursing staff and medical students, as confirmed by recent studies in Australia,[17] Canada[18] and the UK.[19] If directed at students, it can be a cause of considerable distress. Australian hospitals and other institutions are now more aware that bullying occurs in health care and health care education and are beginning to embrace efforts to minimise its incidence and assist those who are targeted. For students bullying can take the form of being shouted at, demeaned in front of others, or being pushed into taking on tasks for which you are not trained. If you feel that you are being bullied, you should discuss the situation with a senior staff member responsible for your medical course.

Some academics speak of the 'informal curriculum' and 'hidden curriculum' of the medical course. These terms seek to distinguish the formal medical school curriculum from additional ways in which medical students learn. The informal curriculum refers to all the teaching and learning that takes place between teachers and students especially in clinical settings. The hidden curriculum refers to more subtle factors that influence medical students such as the positive and negative role models that clinician-teachers may provide and the general environment of the clinical setting – i.e. the culture of the hospital, general practice or other clinical site in which the student spends time.[20]

There are other types of experiences that may create ethical dilemmas for students. These may include conflict between educational need and patient care need such as being asked to perform an examination or procedure not necessary for the care of a patient, being asked to take on responsibilities beyond your current capacity, or witnessing substandard care.[21] You may find these experiences difficult to deal with. Discussing the experience with peers and/or mentors and taking the experience to class discussions on ethics and professionalism can be helpful.[22]

It has become quite common for medical schools to expect that students will learn the techniques of physical examination by practising on fellow students. In some medical schools, students practise simple procedures on each other, under supervision, such as insertion of a needle into a vein. These can be valuable experiences in helping you appreciate what patients go through. However, submitting yourself to be examined by another student or having such a procedure done could be unacceptable to you for a range of reasons. These situations may be distressing even if the medical school allows students to opt out of these activities without 'losing face' or being discriminated against.[23] Medical schools should have written policies about peer physical examinations.[24] Medical school leaders will probably be aware of the gender, cultural and religious issues that can arise for medical students but not all teachers have the same insights. If you are placed in unacceptable situation, you should approach a senior member of the medical school faculty (staff).

A study from New Zealand reported that a small proportion of medical students practise some procedures, including venepuncture and arterial puncture, on themselves in unsupervised and unsafe circumstances and at times unsupported by a fellow medical student.[25] In my view, this is dangerous, unwise and probably unethical. It does not augur well for the sense of professionalism of these students.

Medical students and new medical graduates need to learn about the roles of the other health professionals that they will eventually work with – nurses, pharmacists, physiotherapists and the like. Increasingly the care of patients with complex health problems is delivered by teams composed of a range of health professionals with different skills. Doctors need to learn how to work effectively and cooperatively in such teams. In recognition of the need for mutual understanding of roles as well as effective teamwork, many medical schools have introduced joint learning experiences where medical students and other health care students learn together.

3.6 Can I study medicine and still manage my young family?

Raising a family is not incompatible with undertaking and successfully and happily completing a medical degree and the intern year. However, combining a demanding course such as medicine with having a family clearly creates additional stresses, not only for the medical student but also for the partner of the student. If you are considering this path, you will need to be reasonably secure that you have in place the supports needed. Both you and your partner should be aware of the pressures you will need to cope with.

This subject has been little written about in Australia, perhaps because until quite recently all medical courses were undergraduate of five- or six-years duration and the typical first year student was a school leaver. Some students did marry during the medical course but these were a small minority. Most studies of the difficulties faced by medical students who have partners and who also have children have been undertaken in the USA where graduate entry courses and older medical students are the norm. What follows is drawn predominantly from those studies and extrapolation of any findings to the Australian context may not always be justified.

These 'medical marriages' have been identified by Gerber in his US study[26] as having potential difficulties in the areas of 'specialness', work and study pressures, time pressures and insufficient energy for caring at home. Specialness is the term Gerber used to portray a situation where the medical student's needs for time for clinical experience and for study as well as for financial support are given priority over any needs, emotional or otherwise, of the spouse/partner, as the couple have agreed that the student is engaged in the very special task of becoming a doctor. Most young couples who choose this approach view the situation as a short term challenge that will soon be in the past and that all will be well in the future. Gradually as the student years flow into the equally demanding intern and later training years and then into the difficult years of establishing independent practice, the anticipated happy future of time together as a family never arrives and the partner who sacrificed his or her own career and personal development to support the special medical student may feel as though she or he has been misused or exploited. Gerber's work was published many years ago and thus its relevance to today's medical students is uncertain.

The pressures and demands on a conscientious and ambitious medical student who is striving to keep up with his or her study load can leave little time for a normal family relationship. The hours of study and work can also make it very difficult for the student who is a parent of a young child to have anything more than brief contact with the child during the working week. Should the other partner in the relationship also be studying or be working in a career with long hours of work and similar pressures, these difficulties are compounded. Lack of energy at the end of each demanding day means that time for talking, supporting and caring for each other and any children is also compromised. Feelings of guilt or of anger are quite common. Couples do survive and thrive through these years, especially if they are aware of what lies ahead, are able to openly discuss their genuine feelings and needs, have sufficient supports in place and are capable of making compromises. One of the more difficult compromises for many medical students is the notion of studying a little less conscientiously and accepting 'average' academic results, and thus perhaps having to accept narrower career opportunities, in return for time to develop healthy and rewarding family relationships.

The supports needed vary from couple to couple but may include access to child care, belonging to a discussion/support group of colleagues and friends in similar positions, and finding mentors and supervisors who are understanding, flexible and supportive. Single parents are likely to need even more support. While every medical course is full time, it is always possible to take a year off away from studies without penalty. Taking this opportunity may be one way of reducing the risk to your relationship and providing a better balanced approach to all the competing pressures.

3.7 What are some of the issues for persons with disabilities when studying medicine?

Disabilities come in different forms. The disability of being a healthy carrier of certain viral infections, particularly hepatitis B, has already been mentioned (Section 2.14) and is discussed in depth in Section 4.8. Other disabilities might include problems with eyesight, hearing, or physical mobility and dexterity. The key issues for any prospective medical student with a disability relate to (a) the capacity of the medical school to accommodate the individual's particular disability and (b) the potential impact of the disability on the individual's capacity to complete all the requirements of the medical course as well as on the capacity to complete an intern year to the satisfaction of the Medical Board of Australia. Less importantly, the disability might narrow the fields of medical practice open to one's future career: e.g. being wheelchair-bound would not prevent a successful career as a medical administrator or a psychiatrist but would preclude a career as a surgeon. Medical Deans Australia New Zealand[27] and most medical schools have developed statements about the inherent requirements for the study of medicine which are available on their web sites. People with a disability who wish to study medicine should seek individual advice from a medical school. Students who become disabled during the medical course should also seek advice.

3.8 What if I find part way through my medical course that I don't like it?

This does happen to a small number of students. Admitting to oneself that a wrong choice has been made is not an easy thing to do at any stage of life. Sometimes the warning signs that you are not happy may be overlooked, ignored or given a different explanation. These signs might include missing classes and lectures, struggling to prepare for examinations, or failing them through lack of preparation, and over-involving oneself in non-curricular activities of the university. Should your choice of studying medicine have been influenced by family expectations and pressure, your situation may be even more difficult. If you are having doubts, you should seek independent advice and counselling sooner rather than later. You may also be helped by reading a new book by UK occupational psychologist Caroline Elton.[28]

It is possible that your concerns about finishing the medical course might be surmountable with additional support and wise counsel. Advice is available through university counselling services or directly from senior staff of the medical school, particularly from the local head of your hospital-based clinical school, most often given the title of clinical dean. This position is usually occupied by an experienced doctor whose role encompasses medical student support and well-being; these people are familiar with the difficulties faced by medical students. It might also be important to seek a medical assessment in case your feelings are due to a treatable problem such as a depressive illness.

Depending on the point you have reached in your course and the subjects you have already successfully completed, credit for those subjects may be able to be transferred to a different degree course. If after taking advice you are still unsure of what might be your best option, you should consider requesting a year's deferment from your course to give you time to look at other options and to make your decision under less time pressure.

3.9 How long will I have to study before I get a job?

The length of a medical course ranges from 4 to 6 years but the 4-year courses are 'graduate entry' so a minimum of three years of undergraduate study has to be added on to these 4 years. Courses that enrol school leavers are 5 or 6 years in length. The first salaried 'job' for all graduates is the 'intern' year, also referred to as post graduate year 1 (PGY1). During the intern year, new graduates practise under provisional registration granted by the Medical Board of Australia, a form of registration that involves close supervision, support and ongoing education. The work and training in PGY1 is predominantly undertaken in a hospital setting. At the completion of the intern year and subject to satisfactory supervisor reports, the Medical Board of Australia can grant full (general) registration. Career paths beyond the intern year, and the terminology of hospital and general practice training posts, are discussed in Section 5.

The intern year is not the end of the average doctor's training. Whether one aims to be a family/general practitioner or a specialist of some other type, there will be a number of further years of training, study, theoretical and clinical examinations, and a gradually decreasing level of supervision with a matching increase in level of responsibility and skills. This additional training before independent practice is possible will take six or more years after the intern year. This training is addressed in more detail in Section 5.

Nearly all of this training is undertaken in full time salaried positions in hospitals, or in family practices as a salaried general practice 'registrar' and the salaries increase according to the years of training and the level of responsibility. Job sharing arrangements are increasingly possible but naturally this lengthens the duration of training. Job sharing may be complex to arrange as it requires an available second person, a willing employer and understanding supervisors. The junior doctor training years can be very stressful as they necessarily combine the demands of clinical work, including some shift/night work, with the pressures of finding time to study (see Section 5).

3.10 Are there any other considerations?

Registration of medical students

Under national legislation, all medical students are required to be registered with the Medical Board of Australia (MBA). Student registration is free and individual students are not required to apply for registration. Instead every accredited medical school provides the relevant details of their enrolled students to the MBA each year. The student register held by the MBA is not accessible to the public and any information on that register remains confidential.[29]

Under the national law, the MBA is empowered only to deal with notifications received where (a) a student's health might be so impaired that there may be a risk to the public or (b) a student has been found guilty of an offence punishable by 12 months imprisonment. The MBA thus has no role in handling student performance or misconduct issues. These are the province of the university as discussed below. In the unlikely event that your conduct or your health is the subject of a notification to the MBA, you should seek advice from your medical school or a medical defence organisation.

Student indemnity insurance

It is possible for a medical student to cause harm to a patient and be sued for damages. Because of this slight risk, medical schools arrange for insurance to cover this possibility, at no cost to students. Some medical schools also advise their students to join a medical indemnity organisation as this is free until graduation, when it becomes a requirement for medical registration.

Student misconduct and unprofessional behaviour

In Section 1, the qualities expected of a good doctor were listed and they included honesty and truthfulness. As medical student misconduct and unprofessional behaviour have been identified as harbingers of professional misconduct after graduation leading to disciplinary actions by medical registration boards[30] it should come as no surprise that medical schools take student misconduct very seriously. Academic misconduct includes cheating at examinations, submitting work that is not one's own, forging signatures, and plagiarism. Other serious forms of misconduct include exploiting patients or their families for your own purposes, such as making sexually explicit remarks or sexual overtures to patients, making racist or sexist remarks to patients, and showing disrespect to patients, teachers, clinicians and fellow students. Unprofessional behaviours have been categorised into four groups: failure to engage, dishonest behaviour, disrespectful behaviour, and poor self-awareness.[31] Unprofessional student behaviour in the US study of Papadakis and colleagues included irresponsibility, diminished capacity for self-improvement, immaturity and poor initiative. These were often accompanied by lack of insight and resistance to suggested improvement. In the same study, doctors who had been disciplined by a medical board were more likely while in medical school to have demonstrated impaired relationships with peers, teachers and nursing staff, and unprofessional behaviour associated with being nervous, anxious or insecure.

Misuse of legal drugs, including alcohol and prescription only drugs, and use of illegal drugs such as marijuana and cocaine by medical students also predicts later problems for those students when they engage in the rigours of clinical practice. Most Australian medical schools have established what have been called 'fitness to practise' policies along with disciplinary and remediation pathways. These policies address a range of conduct issues including: criminal conviction or caution; drug or alcohol misuse; aggressive, violent or threatening behaviour; cheating or plagiarising; dishonesty or fraud; unprofessional behaviour or attitudes, including inappropriate use of social media; and health concerns, as well as seeking to develop student insight into and appropriate management of these conduct issues.[32] At present, other than where a student's alleged misconduct may impose a risk to patients, that conduct is an internal matter for the medical school and does not have to be reported to the medical board.[33]

The use and misuse of alcohol can be problematic for medical students. The sense of camaraderie among medical students and the numerous social functions at university, commonly arranged by the medical students' society, mean that the risk of excessive intake of alcohol is ever present. Drinking patterns established at this stage can persist for a lifetime, especially if alcohol is being used to cope with stress, anxiety or depression during the medical course.

The issue of professional misconduct by doctors is discussed in Section 5, Attachment A.

3.11 Applying to be registered after graduation

All medical graduates must undertake an intern year before being eligible for full medical registration. Prior to commencing the intern year, new graduates are granted provisional registration with the Medical Board of Australia. Each medical school provides the state office of the MBA with the details of all its new graduates and provides those graduates with information about the steps required to gain provisional registration. Under national law, it is now necessary for each applicant for initial registration to produce a statement from the police regarding the absence of any criminal record (a 'police check'). It is also necessary to meet the strict English language standards for registration as a doctor; where there is doubt, formal testing of language ability may be required.

3.12 When should I start thinking about my career beyond graduation?

Only a minority of medical students graduate with very firm ideas about the type of medical career they will pursue. Many students report having some intentions at this point (often based on satisfying time spent as a student in a particular area of general practice, a hospital based term in medicine, surgery, paediatrics or a time with other services) only to change their mind after further good experiences during the intern year and second post-graduate year (PGY2).

The first decision about the general direction of one's career comes part way through the intern year. At this point, you will need to decide on the type of experience you hope to have in PGY2. Most hospitals offer combinations of four or five 10–14-week rotations in year 2 through both hospital and external placements designed to suit broad career paths, viz. the paths to general practice, surgery, medicine or critical care (critical care covers intensive care, emergency medicine and anaesthetics). However, this decision is by no means final and many young doctors change career choices during PGY2, or in PGY3, without great disadvantage. Beyond that time, because of the requirements of the medical colleges (see Section 5), it becomes more difficult to change direction without effectively 'losing' or repeating a year of training.

The topic of how to think through career options is discussed in more detail in Section 5. During the PGY1 and PGY2 years, virtually all medical graduates will have a home base of a teaching hospital. These institutions employ medical staff as directors of training supported by medical educators so that ready sources of advice about career options will be available to you.

THE REALITY OF LIFE AS A MEDICAL STUDENT

Most medical students enjoy their experience overall. However, some find parts of the course stressful. In this section, I provide advice about aspects that are likely to be challenging, how to cope with stresses, and where assistance may be sought. Advice is also provided about approach to study and about maintaining a healthy lifestyle.

4.1 What is it like to be a medical student?

Very few accounts have been written about the lives of medical students* in Australia so this section is based on past student experiences, input from current and recent Australian students and an interpretation of published experiences from elsewhere.

The AME Study of 2005–7 mentioned earlier asked medical students and recent medical graduates (interns) about their experiences and 79% of those surveyed were satisfied or very satisfied with their overall medical education and their preparedness for the intern year.[1] So the first message is that despite the demands of the medical course, most students cope well, enjoy the experience and go on to be contented competent doctors. But it is not true for all students as a proportion of students are at times

---

* While written accounts are sparse, a wide variety of experiences can be found on the internet such as this one: https://www.youtube.com/watch?v=nsH81_P4Obk.

unduly stressed by their experiences. Even so, most of these distressed students graduate and enjoy successful careers somewhere in medicine. What follows is focussed on some of the more common causes of stress and distress among medical students and how these pressures can be best managed.

4.2 How demanding is the medical course?

All medical courses place substantial demands on their students. Every course is full time and courses are crowded with tasks including tutorials, lectures, preparing for group work such as case-based learning, team-based learning or problem-based learning, assessing patients (clerking) and progress examinations. Most segments of every course have attendance requirements that need to be satisfied. Clinical placements, which may be distant and even interstate, can require significant time commitments of students, which may include times normally regarded as after hours. These placements will need flexibility in regard to hours of attendance and may test your physical and mental stamina. Some rural placements may require a driving licence and a roadworthy vehicle.

There is a lot to learn, remember and understand but many of the demands of the course relate more to the organisation and use of your time than to any intellectual pressure. So long as you have the capacity to apply yourself steadily to the demands of the course, are not too distracted by outside demands (including part time work), and do not suffer any health issues, you should be confident of completing the course. The phrase 'not too distracted by outside demands' has been chosen deliberately as it is equally important to maintain a healthy social life, to keep up other interests, hobbies or physical or sporting activities, and remain a part of the broader Australian community.

Getting the balance right between study and life at this stage forms important preparation for the later demands of medical practice. Learning how to be fully focussed on the task at hand, your studies now but later the patient in front of you, and yet to be able to put work behind you in your leisure time and family time will be invaluable in coping with the demands of being a doctor.

From time to time, one will read about medical students and new medical graduates who have been able to combine the efforts involved in completing the medical course with other pursuits that also involve devoted study or training. These people have achieved success for example as musicians or as sportspeople as well as graduating as doctors, thus indicating that it is possible to avoid making medical studies the only focus of one's life.

4.3 What do students say are the most enjoyable parts of the course?

In contrast to many other university courses, medical students spend large amounts of time together in large and small groups on the main university campus, at hospitals and in other clinical settings. This, together with the sharing of new, stressful or unique experiences (e.g. dissecting a human cadaver), usually fosters a great sense of camaraderie among the student body leading to many lifelong friendships. Students also enjoy the privilege of spending time with patients and learning from them. These experiences together with the knowledge that a satisfying career is not too far away makes the medical course a very rewarding and enjoyable experience for most but not all students. In the AME Study, 87% of Australian junior doctors were either satisfied or very satisfied with their overall medical education.[2]

4.4 Is the course stressful and what aspects might be stressful?

The majority of recent graduates are able to recall some aspects of their course that were stressful. Most students at some time feel overwhelmed by the amount of new knowledge that they are expected to acquire and are apprehensive about their capacity to cope with the study load. These stresses are compounded by assessments and examinations. Other sources of stress include dealing with death or suffering, interactions with teachers, new methods of learning including presenting cases, talking with patients with severe mental illness, lack of control over workload and demands, and observing questionable performances of doctors.[3] Late in any course, concerns over finding a suitable intern position may also cause stress, especially for international students who are not guaranteed these places (see Section 5).

There are reports of students being stressed by exposure to poor conduct towards themselves or fellow students such as humiliation by teachers, junior doctors or nurses, discrimination on the grounds of gender or ethnicity, or sexual advances by teachers or supervisors.[4] In a study from New Zealand,[5] two thirds of medical students reported adverse experiences, the most common being the experience of humiliation, but also included unfair treatment based on gender or race and unwanted sexual advances. The authors commented that humiliation had an adverse effect on learning.

Some students feel extremely uncomfortable with the task of dissecting cadavers as part of the study of human anatomy. Close contact with a seriously ill and dying patient, especially if the patient is of similar age to you or has an illness that has also affected a close friend or family member can also be very distressing. Medical students who have experienced the death of a parent are particularly likely to find clinical contact with seriously ill and dying patients emotionally disturbing.

In this environment, if you are unfortunate enough to also experience a serious stress in your private life, as for example a death in your family or a breakdown of a long term relationship, you are likely to find aspects of your course more burdensome than usual.

Other students may be stressed by financial issues such as the cost of the course, debt and anticipated debt or by the demands of trying to fit in part time work with a medical school study program. Temporary relocation for distant clinical rotations may also be stressful, through their impact on relationships or on part time work.[6]

The impact of any stresses experienced is likely to vary according to the temperament, personal situation and vulnerabilities of each medical student. Personal predictors of distress include perfectionism, self-criticism and feelings of being an impostor[7] and the traits of neuroticism and conscientiousness.[8] On the other hand conscientiousness is a predictor of good performance in medical school, especially when combined with sociability (extraversion, openness, good self-esteem). Conscientiousness however may be a problem if combined with neuroticism.[9]

How stressful any experiences may be are not only related to individual vulnerabilities but also to the leadership of, and support offered through the culture of, any particular medical school. Medical schools that offer smaller teaching/learning groups where the composition of the small group is stable over time appear to have happier and less stressed students.[10]

Burnout, defined as feelings of emotional exhaustion, depersonalisation and/or reduced feelings of personal accomplishment, has also been reported in significant proportions of medical students, particularly in the USA where all students undertake four year graduate entry medical courses and are expected to spend more time in hospital wards and with more responsibilities than do Australian students. Burnout has been less extensively studied in Australian medical students but with the move to shorter duration graduate entry courses, the risk may be higher. A 2004 Australian study of final year medical students from a new graduate entry medical course reported symptoms consistent with burnout in 28%.[11] A 2016 study of year 1 and year 2 students at Australian UG and GE courses reported burnout in 50% of both groups of students.[12] These findings were confirmed in 2016 study at another graduate entry course which reported high levels of anxiety and stress, with levels being higher in older students.[13]

Tearfulness in relation to contact with patients, most often in the context of suffering and/or dying patients is also quite common.[14] One American study of crying among medical students linked crying to the presence of symptoms of burnout.[15]

It has also been suggested by Benbassat and colleagues that medical students and doctors in training are ill-prepared for some aspects of student and medical life and that this lack of preparation should be seen as an additional stressor needing attention. For example, students are surprised to find that doctors have to function with much greater uncertainty than the students had imagined, and that such uncertainty may at times translate inappropriately into feelings of personal inadequacy. This lack of preparation may be compounded when, after leaving the teaching hospital environment, new doctors find that the biomedical model of ill-health has not equipped them well for the problems they commonly encounter that are driven by psycho-social factors. The authors propose that this stressor as well as all other common stressors be realistically addressed during training and that it be made clear that professional distress for students and doctors is 'pervasive rather than due to individual inadequacies'.[16] Benbassat has also pointed out that the medical learning environment may contribute to the poor preparation of students through denial of uncertainty in clinical medicine, belittling of students, and failing to reduce the stigma of mental ill-health, and has called for a more nurturing attitude such that students are regarded as junior colleagues.[17]

The Australian Medical Students' Association has joined forces with the New Zealand Medical Students' Association to produce a detailed 'wellbeing guide' for medical students entitled 'Keeping Your Grass Greener'.[18] This contains a large amount of very useful advice from a range of experts covering such aspects as preventing and managing burnout and stress. It also provides contact details for sources of help available for distressed medical students in every Australian state and territory and in New Zealand.

4.5 The consequences of burnout and prevention of burnout

Burnout can be associated with anxiety and depression and has been linked to feelings of reduced altruism, diminished empathy with patients[19] and suicidal thoughts.[20] In addition, burnout has been linked to student misconduct including cheating, plagiarism and other misdemeanours, perhaps in response to stressed students looking for 'shortcuts' when overwhelmed by workloads.[21]

Feelings of burnout can be reduced if the learning environment is positive and supportive.[22] Some Australian medical schools are now trialling new programs to assist students to learn self-care skills to better cope with stresses in the medical course and to prepare them for the stresses of medical practice.[23]

You can reduce the risk of burnout by a number of approaches including seeking support from peers and mentors, allocating adequate time to social and personal life,[24] taking advice on study, learning methods and time management, ensuring adequate rest, relaxation and physical activity, and seeking confidential professional help if stress levels are high or symptoms of burnout appear. To this list the Australian Medical Students' Association adds maintaining a good diet, avoiding excessive alcohol use and having your own GP.[25]

As discussed below in the context of depression, you might be reluctant to admit that you need help for possible burnout because of fear of stigmatisation. Having a supportive peer group with whom you can discuss yours concerns openly is one starting point. If or when you do approach one of the recommended sources of professional help, you will find that you are not alone.

4.6 Does stress affect the health of medical students?

Medical students in Australia and elsewhere have been reported to experience a range of health issues, including burnout, anxiety and depression, probably related primarily to the stresses of their medical course. These stresses may be contributed to by financial pressures, social isolation or relationship issues. As described above, another source of stress can be the behaviour of teachers and other health professionals.

From my time as chair of the Board of the Victorian Doctors Health Program, I am aware that of the 150 or so new clients seen each year, about a quarter were distressed and unwell medical students while about a third were young doctors in training. By far the commonest problems for the medical students were symptoms ascribable to stress and anxiety, but some students were clinically depressed and a few students with drug and/or alcohol misuse were seen. The range of problems in the medical students and the doctors in training had much in common, suggesting that health issues in student years may be harbingers of later problems and deserve to be managed actively.

Similar experiences have been reported from Norway where 17% of medical students were assessed as having mental health problems in need of treatment, although few had sought help.[26] More recently, a national survey of the mental health of Australian medical students and doctors conducted for the national organisation Beyond Blue[27] reported that 18% of medical students had been diagnosed with depression, many reported anxiety and emotional exhaustion and that one in five had thought about suicide. The response rate to the survey was 27% of the 42,942 doctors and 6,658 medical students who were approached so it is difficult to know the exact size of the mental health issues; they may well be more common. The survey confirmed that doctors and students were concerned at the stigmatisation of mental ill-health.

A study from Canada in 2016 also reported that some students suffered high levels of psychological distress and that this was linked to substance misuse, depression and suicidal ideation.[28] The authors importantly noted that of their students around half sought help from a family doctor. However, many of these students presented with, i.e. complained of, only physical symptoms and unless the doctor probed for emotional issues, the cause of the symptoms may not have become apparent immediately. A 2019 review of world experience found that the pooled prevalence of depression in medical students was 27%.[29]

Depression can be a very difficult issue for medical students. The Beyond Blue survey and surveys from the USA show that medical students are reluctant to seek help through fear of being stigmatised by their fellow students and fear that their teachers might not trust them with responsibilities.[30] In Australia, medical students have access to confidential medical services that are independent of and separate from their medical teachers, as discussed in the next section. These services are very aware of the issue of stigmatisation and take confidentiality very seriously. Students who sense they are unwell or depressed should not hesitate to seek this confidential assistance.

4.7 Is help readily available if I am stressed or unwell?

Yes, all universities are aware of and alert to the fact that students can become unwell or stressed and anxious or depressed and that if not helped, may suffer personally and academically. All universities have established health services that provide confidential assistance to students and most have separate counselling services for students who experience difficulties unrelated to their health. A number of senior staff in medical schools are available to support students, in particular the associate dean or head of the clinical school in your hospital, as well as senior staff who agree to participate in mentoring programs for individual students.

A survey of Australian and New Zealand medical students conducted by medical students and reported in 2010[31] showed that most medical students were aware of the support services at their university but over half of those surveyed believed there was a stigma attached to seeking help for stress or distress. Some medical schools, recognising this stigma, encourage medical students to seek help off campus, such as via the doctors' health advisory services established in each state and territory. For example Victoria has its Victorian Doctors Health Program[32] while NSW has its Doctors' Health Advisory Service (DHAS).[33] These and similar programs in the other states accept and assist medical students. The NSW DHAS website provides links to the services in those states and territories.[34]

The Australian Medical Students Association publication *Keeping Your Grass Greener: A Wellbeing Guide for Medical Students*[35] also contains a detailed list of services and resources available to distressed students. The guide emphasises the importance and value of every student having a general practitioner and suggests ways of finding a GP who is interested in and capable of caring for medical students and fellow doctors.

4.8 Are there any other risks to my own health?

In general, medical students are not as exposed to risks to their health and wellbeing as are doctors and other health professionals who directly care for patients. The most commonly recognised risk to health is the transmission of infections from patients to health care workers, especially of blood borne viruses (HIV, hepatitis B and hepatitis C) that may be accidentally transmitted, usually by 'needlestick' injury. Students should not be expected to undertake procedures on patients known to carry such infections, but these risks do not disappear after graduation (unless a non-clinical career path is chosen). A number of other potentially serious infectious diseases can be spread by droplet (coughing, sneezing) via the respiratory tract, as for example influenza and tuberculosis. Medical students are not placed knowingly in settings that carry such risk but, on the other hand, a student may be asked to see a newly admitted patient in whom the diagnosis is not yet known.

Newly emerging but still rare infectious diseases for which no treatments are available (e.g. Ebola virus, avian influenza) create ethical dilemmas when doctors, nurses and others are expected to care for patients with such diseases. It is not clear that health care workers can be conscripted into such work. Understandably, other serious responsibilities, for example duties to spouse and children, might make a doctor or a nurse feel reluctant to undertake such work. However, the recent history is that doctors and nurses rarely shirk such duties. By seeking to join the medical profession in clinical work, you are tacitly accepting this ethical obligation.

Before enrolling in a medical course, students are required to receive vaccinations to prevent a range of illnesses. From an early stage of their studies they are given education about minimising risks of contracting infections and of spreading infections. The committee of deans of Australian and New Zealand medical schools, known officially as Medical Deans Australia New Zealand, has developed and published best practice guidelines covering what is required of medical schools to meet their duty of care towards students and patients.[36] Patients can be put at risk by students with infections transmissible to others as discussed below. The guidelines emphasise that medical schools should provide a copy of the school's policies and procedures about infectious diseases to each student prior to their enrolling. In brief, these guidelines cover the legal duty of medical schools to ensure the safety of students and patients, the need to have clear and enforced policies that distinguish between the responsibilities to its students and responsibilities to patients that students have contact with, a requirement that medical students are fully informed about the policies and give informed consent to the application of those policies, details of any vaccination/ immunisation requirements, the choice of opting out of immunisation for medical or conscience grounds and details of requirements for screening tests for certain transmissible diseases. These policies are usually available on medical school web sites. In addition there are national guidelines for all health care workers that are updated regularly.[37]

The Medical Deans' guidelines address issues of confidentiality of screening test results and limitations as to who is permitted or required to be informed about a positive test. They also advise on access for students to expert advice from an infectious diseases specialist if needed. The medical school is expected to cover the cost of any tests and vaccinations and to provide academic, personal and career counselling for students with blood-borne viruses and other infectious diseases. Attachments to the guidelines list all the infectious diseases for which immunisation is required and provide detailed instructions about testing for and responding to tests for blood-borne viruses (i.e. HIV, hepatitis B and hepatitis C).

The most immediately relevant aspect of screening for transmissible diseases is the reality that a small number of medical students are healthy carriers of the blood-borne virus, hepatitis B. In these instances, they are likely to have been infected at birth. This occurs very rarely now for Australian born infants but still happens in some developing countries. There are degrees of infectivity among those infected with hepatitis B as measured by viral load. Thus some carriers of the virus are deemed to pose sufficient risk to patients that they are not permitted to undertake exposure prone medical procedures.* There are a large number of areas of clinical medicine that do not involve doctors undertaking exposure prone procedures so a medical career is still very possible for carriers of hepatitis B. However, in the compulsory provisional registration year (intern year – see below), some rotations such as to surgery and emergency departments do involve exposure prone procedures. Interns with infectious diseases will need to have their intern experience modified, consistent with national guidelines and guided by an infectious diseases specialist who will liaise with the employing hospital(s).

Most medical schools offer elective clinical experiences overseas and some of these may be to countries where certain infectious diseases (e.g. HIV, TB or malaria) are common. Medical schools will provide students with individual advice ahead of such travel and it is essential that students seek out and heed such advice.

Before leaving the topic of infectious diseases, the possibility of students spreading more common infections to the patients they come into contact with needs to be recognised. The guidelines mentioned above cover the need for medical student to be immunised against common infections (e.g. pertussis, measles and varicella) that if passed on to ill and immunologically compromised patients might be fatal. Students who are ill with infectious diseases such as influenza should avoid close contact with

---

*   Exposure prone procedures are internationally defined as a subset of invasive procedures that involve potential direct contact between the skin of the doctor (most often the thumb or a finger) and a sharp instruments or sharp tissues such as bone spicules, usually during a procedure undertaken in a confined or poorly visualised anatomic site, including the oral cavity.

patients while they remain infectious. This is one part of 'patient safety', a very important element of the professional responsibilities of doctors which will be covered during your training.

As mentioned in Section 2.5, medical students receive instruction in hand hygiene and are expected to comply with rigorous practices to prevent cross infection. It has been estimated that there are over 80,000 hospital acquired infections in Australia per year, and doctors and students share the challenge in reducing these numbers.[38] It is easy to know when you are sick, but only routine optimal hand hygiene habits will help prevent the transmission of microscopic germs from patient to patient by contaminated hands. Unfortunately you will certainly observe that experienced doctors can be poor role models in this matter.[39]

Another potential source of harm is from physical violence. Students are rarely exposed to physical harm from disturbed and violent patients but again it needs to be recognised by prospective doctors that in Australia, from time to time, doctors and other health care professionals are at risk of physical violence from disturbed or drug affected patients and a small number have been fatally harmed by patients.

4.9 Tips for success as a medical student

How you care for yourself and the manner in which you approach getting the right balance between study and other aspects of your life is very important, not only for success and enjoyment of your student days but also because this will help you develop a similar balanced approach to your professional life and the practice of medicine. No matter how hard you feel you need to study at various points during your medical course, it is vital that you also make time for recreation, be it music, sport, reading or some other hobby or interest, and for maintaining your circle of friends. A sensible lifestyle should also include time allocated for physical exercise, adequate and regular nutrition and adequate sleep.

For most students, the medical course is a challenge primarily because of the large amount of new information that needs to be understood and remembered. It has been said that it takes a vocabulary of around 3,000 words to be fluent in another language and that in becoming a doctor students learn up to 6,000 new words! Very few students fail subjects during the course but those who do are most likely to have been disorganised and erratic in their approach to study, perhaps because they were distracted by other things or were stressed and unwell. You need to think about what study methods work best for you.

Some things just have to be learnt by heart and most students sensibly use mnemonics to assist where possible. Another learning technique that works well for most students is to write things down when revising from lecture notes or textbooks, instead of just reading them. If you are lucky enough to have a photographic memory then enjoy your luck. Others will summarise material from lectures into point form lists, on cards or stored electronically, more easily and quickly revised before examinations. Whatever approach you take, you will be wise to be systematic, consistent and regular in your study habits.

Some students like to join a study group with fellow students as this will provide mutual support and help you gauge where your knowledge levels are at. Study groups may evolve from PBL groups or from groups allocated to clinical rotations in later years of the course. However, a study group may not suit your learning style and not all study groups function efficiently, so don't feel that this is essential. If you are confident about your capacity for self-directed and self-motivated learning, a study group may be of less benefit to you. All the above issues about learning at medical school are addressed in detail in a book written for UK medical students.[40] Much of its content is relevant for, and is likely to be of assistance to, Australian medical students.

A very important goal of your training is to be competent in eliciting the history of a patient and conducting a physical examination of that patient. Both of these skills are learned and do not come naturally so every opportunity to see and learn from patients should be grasped. These opportunities are mostly available during the normal working week, so during your clinical training years, if you need to also be working part-time to support yourself, you should avoid if possible part-time work during the weekdays.

As already discussed, surveys here and abroad indicate that up to a quarter of medical students can experience stress and distress, so you need to be alert to your own feelings and emotions. Sharing your feelings with close friends who are also students may help you assess yourself. If you are feeling anxious or are not sleeping well, you should seek advice, available from your own general practitioner, from the university student health service or from an independent doctors' health service in your state. This can be a time when dangerous practices are tempting, including self –medication with excess amounts of alcohol or with medicines obtained from misguided friends and colleagues. For many of those doctors whose careers are later blighted by substance abuse, misuse commenced during their student days.

The Australian Medical Students' Association with the New Zealand Medical Students' Association have published *Keeping Your Grass Greener: A Wellbeing Guide for Medical Students*.[41] It could usefully be read by all medical students as it contains a great deal of practical advice about preventing and coping with the various stresses of the medical course.

THE INTERN YEAR AND BEYOND: CAREER PATHS FOR MEDICAL GRADUATES

For medical students nearing the completion of their medical course, the main focus is on what happens in the intern year. In this section I provide advice about what the intern year entails and about caring for oneself during this year. The section also covers how to apply for an internship, the process of medical registration and the implications of being a registered medical practitioner. In addition, the section provides a summary of career pathways, guidance as to where more detailed information about career options may be found and advice about choosing a suitable field of practice.

5.1 What is the intern year and what does it entail?

The first year after completing your medical course is the intern year, also known as postgraduate year 1 (PGY1). All medical graduates must satisfactorily* complete an accredited intern year before they can be granted

---

* This means that your progress reports provided by your allocated term supervisor for each rotation during your intern year must be satisfactory. The report form is standardised across most of the nation and supervisors are asked to rate your performance under a series of headings including patient assessment, patient

full, i.e. general, medical registration. The intern year must include at least 47 weeks of full-time work. Although unusual, it is possible to negotiate a job-sharing arrangement such that the requirements of the intern year can be completed over two years.[1] All resident Australians who graduate from Australian medical schools are currently guaranteed an intern position and this is unlikely to change in the foreseeable future. Until recently, all international graduates of Australian medical schools were usually able to obtain an intern position if they sought one. However, the expansion of medical schools together with an increase in the number of international students enrolling in the courses means that intern positions in Australia now may not be available to all international students who graduate here.

While an intern/provisional registration year is a feature common to most developed countries, the nature of the experience offered varies widely. In Australia, the emphasis is on a broad experience across medicine, surgery, emergency medical care and other fields. In some other countries, the intern year is quite specialised and the new graduate is asked to choose an internship year spent entirely in an area such as psychiatry, surgery, family medicine, a medical speciality or paediatrics.

The intern year is a vitally important transition year where the graduating medical student moves into the role of formally caring for and treating patients. The nature of the work you will do and the rotations and level of ongoing education and support provided to you is subject to the intern positions offered being accredited by the postgraduate education council* of your state or territory. The intern year is meant to combine education and training with service provision but on some rotations and

---

safety, patient management, communication, use of investigations, prescribing, performing procedures and information management. You will be asked to make a self-assessment during each rotation and the clinical supervisor will meet with you to discuss and complete the report.

* Postgraduate education councils, or their equivalent, exist in all jurisdictions. For example, in NSW, the body is named the Health Education and Training Institute. These councils are responsible for visiting and accrediting the hospitals and other organisations that employ interns. In turn, these councils are accredited for their role by the Australian Medical Council, a process designed to ensure similar standards of training, education and support for interns throughout Australia.

in some hospitals, service demands may be overwhelming. You will now be paid a reasonable salary; in January 2019 annual intern salaries ranged from $67,950 in NSW to $78,479 in Western Australia.[2] With most employment contracts, you are entitled to claim for overtime worked but you may find that your employing hospital does not encourage such claims. You will now also begin to repay your HECS/ HELP debt.

As an intern, you will be registered with the Medical Board of Australia* under the category of provisional registration which means that you can only practise under supervision in the accredited rotations in which you will be placed by your employing hospital or hospital network. The rotations must involve ten-week terms each in medicine and surgery and an eight-week term in emergency medical care. Other rotations will be in a variety of clinical settings. The expansion in the number of Australian medical schools has resulted in the need to accredit additional supervised intern positions. This has led to the extension of internship experience into networks of country hospitals, some private hospitals and even general practice, providing interns with a broader exposure to the Australian health care system.

Final year medical students typically feel quite anxious as to whether they have sufficient knowledge or have acquired sufficient practical skills to be able to cope with the start of the intern year. This is a natural feeling even though most medical schools provide 'intern like' experiences (pre-internships) in the last year of the course. Prospective employers and future supervisors would probably be concerned about any new graduate who was supremely confident about his or her abilities! However, a 2005 survey of Australian interns reported that interns generally felt that their training had prepared them well for their intern year, although some understandably still felt a lack of confidence at the start of the year.[3]

More recently the Australian Medical Council together with the Medical Board of Australia has conducted an annual survey of preparedness

---

* The cost of provisional registration in 2019 was $382. After graduating, you will need to remain registered with the MBA until you retire from practice. You should be taught about the role of the Board during your medical course but for readers unfamiliar with the MBA and its role, Attachment A provides a brief summary.

for internship.[4] The proportion of interns who completed the 2017 survey was disappointing at around 20%; hopefully interns in the future will take more interest in it. Nevertheless, of those who responded, 75% agreed that their medical course had prepared them well for internship while only 11% disagreed. The survey was detailed and allowed examination of many subsets of skills and competencies. Interns reported that they felt underprepared for prescribing, coping with uncertainty and reporting errors. Many felt underprepared in non-clinical matters including seeking support for emotional distress for themselves or colleagues and for dealing with harassment or bullying. These findings have been shared with supervisors across the country and with medical schools and should lead to further improvements in the medical course curriculum and in the support and education provided in the intern year – and hence the importance of interns responding to future surveys.

In the second half of 2019, a survey was undertaken of the 30,000 medical trainees, including interns, throughout Australia to ask for the trainees' views on the quality of their training and to seek to 'identify issues that could impact on patient safety, including environment and culture, unacceptable behaviours and the quality of supervision'. The findings, not available at the time of publication, may also lead to improvements in the experience of trainees.[5]

As part of providing accredited intern positions, hospitals are obliged to provide detailed orientation programs, usually of 3–5 days duration, before new interns start work. These programs should provide opportunities to revise and practise the procedures they will be expected to undertake. Throughout the year, interns are supported and supervised by more experienced doctors, usually a registrar (see footnote page 129) as well as a senior consultant. Interns are on a steep learning curve and are *not* expected to know everything or have had extensive hands on experience undertaking procedures on patients. However they do need to demonstrate a preparedness to admit their own knowledge deficits and a willingness to ask questions and to seek support and supervision.

Hospitals nominated as the home base for interns have a senior doctor appointed as director of clinical studies or supervisor of intern training, supported by a dedicated medical education officer. Together their task is to oversee the formal and informal training of interns and ensure that interns and other junior medical staff are adequately supported. Interns should also take responsibility for their own education by asking questions and reading about patients under their care and by attending scheduled training sessions. The Australian Medical Council and the Medical Board of Australia have developed Intern Outcome Statements that state the broad and significant outcomes that interns should achieve by the end of the internship year. Health services that provide internship programs are responsible for designing programs that will allow interns to achieve these outcomes.

It is possible that in the next few years some aspects of the intern year may be altered in response to a national review completed in 2015.[6] Among a range of recommendations, the review suggested that more should be done to expose interns to the 'full patient journey' and not just acute hospital care. This could lead to a compulsory term in some area of community medicine or general practice. It also recommended that a two-year capability and performance framework be developed but with the provisional registration period remaining the first (intern) year. This recommendation and many others have been accepted by Australia's health ministers but it is not yet known when such changes will eventuate. The reviewers were sensitive to the need to not further lengthen the periods of postgraduate training and alert to the value of a broad intern year in helping career planning.

There are a number of additional sources and guidance about the intern year including from the Australian Medical Students Association,[7] the Australian Medical Association,[8] the Australian Medical Council[9] and the Medical Board of Australia.[10]

5.2 How do I seek or find an intern position?

Relevant information will be made available to you during the first half of your final year as a medical student. Through the office of the Australian Health Practitioner Regulation Agency, final year students are allocated a unique identifying number which you will receive via your medical school. This number must be used when applying for an internship. The process of selection is conducted at the state and territory level and is usually managed by the state postgraduate medical council on behalf of the state department of health. As noted, the postgraduate medical council equivalents may have other names in some jurisdictions (see also Table 2).

The method of selection varies between the states and territories, but is usually based on merit and includes a 'computer matching service', allowing you to prioritise the hospitals or hospital networks where you hope to be employed. In general, each jurisdiction gives first priority to graduates of medical schools in that state or territory and lower priority to applicants from interstate or those who are not Australian or New Zealand citizens or Australian permanent residents. In some jurisdictions there are separate pathways to rural internships. These variations mean that you must carefully study the application guide on any relevant website.

Very helpful information is also available through the Australian Medical Students Association internship guide.[11] It notably includes detailed information directed at international medical students who are seeking internships in Australia.

As many final year students apply in more than one state, the jurisdictions cooperate to have a common date for applications to be lodged (usually mid-year). The date of application and the subsequent requirement to promptly respond when you are offered an intern position are rigidly adhered to so it is critical that you carefully note those dates and timings. Table 2 lists the councils and their websites where this information is to be found.

Table 2:
The postgraduate medical councils and their equivalents

ACT	Canberra Region Medical Education Council (CRMEC); http://crmec.health.act.gov.au
NSW	Health Education and Training Institute (HETI); http://www.heti.nsw.gov.au
NT	Northern Territory Prevocational Medical Assurance Service (NT PMAS); http://www.ntmetc.com
QLD	Medical Advisory and Prevocational Accreditation Unit, QLD (MAPAU) (Information about intern positions is accessible at https://www.health.qld.gov.au/employment/work-for-us/clinical/medical/recruitment/intern)
SA	South Australian Medical Education & Training (SAMET); https://www.samet.org.au
TAS	Postgraduate Medical Education Council of Tasmania (PMCT); http://www.pmct.org.au
VIC	Postgraduate Medical Council of Victoria (PMCV); http://www.pmcv.com.au
WA	Postgraduate Medical Council of Western Australia (PMCWA); https://ww2.health.wa.gov.au/About-us/Postgraduate-Medical-Council

Because some students who apply do not graduate, or become ill, or accept an offer overseas, the finalisation of the computer match may be delayed for some applicants and late offers of a place may be made. The intern selection process is overseen and audited by a national committee which issues an audit report each year.[12]

Hospitals generally compete keenly for the 'best' new graduates and hospital representatives may seek to make presentations to your student group or will hold information nights at the hospital, to encourage you to make that hospital your first choice in the matching process. In some states, a whole day is devoted to a 'careers expo' at which most hospitals make staff available to talk to potential interns at a hospital 'booth'. These 'expos' are well advertised to medical students. Information should also be available on your state postgraduate medical council website.[13] Another way of obtaining information about where you might do an internship is to talk to junior doctors a year or two ahead of you. They will know at first-hand what the 'culture' and level of support offered to interns was like in the various rotations they took.

Most hospitals like to interview applicants for intern positions so you will need to give thought to preparing for interviews. One question you are sure to be asked is why you want to spend your intern year at that particular hospital so make sure that you have an answer ready. A practice interview is likely to give you more confidence for the real thing.[14]

5.3 Is the intern year stressful? How can I best deal with this?

Yes, the intern year can be stressful but the stresses experienced by new medical graduates differ somewhat from those experienced by medical students. A 2009 Australian survey of interns reported high levels of stress in 65% and burnout symptoms in 31%. Ninety percent of respondents felt they had been well supported and 82% enjoyed their work.[15] A similar study of interns, residents and registrars reported comparable findings with burnout at 60% while 54% of respondents reported 'compassion fatigue'.[16] Importantly, in both studies nearly a fifth of respondents stated that they would not choose medicine if they started again. A 2004 study of graduates from one Australian medical school also reported high levels of stress and symptoms of burnout in interns.[17] It has sometimes been suggested that burnout symptoms are a reflection of the individual intern's own make-up but this is not the view of one of the world's leading researchers who wrote that 'factors within the learning and work environment, rather than individual attributes, are the major drivers of burnout'.[18]

As the responses to the surveys above were made at a single point in time, it is not known how these particular groups of young doctors felt or will feel about their careers when all their training is completed. Data from a large longitudinal study (MABEL – see Section 1.9) shows high levels of job satisfaction in Australian doctors, including specialists-in-training. Thus it is likely that job satisfaction increases as training progresses or is completed and you have clinical independence and control over your working life. For a small minority of doctors this is not the case and this is discussed below.

The stressful experiences in the first year after graduation include dealing with newly gained responsibility, managing uncertainty, dealing with death and dying, coping with unpredictable workloads, working in multi-profession teams, feeling unsupported, concern about making errors, and the threat or reality of complaints.[19] Lack of feedback about one's performance can also be stressful. Most of these stresses are predictable but the responses of interns are not. Some interns adjust very rapidly to their new professional role while others struggle to come to terms with the workloads and responsibilities and may feel overwhelmed. It is important to realise that such feelings are very common and bear little or no relationship to your eventual competence in your chosen career path. Indeed being so common, discussing your feelings and experiences with fellow interns may help you to cope. However, the feelings can lead to stress and anxiety, and sometimes significant depression. These feelings should not be ignored and you should not hesitate to seek confidential advice. A starting point will be the supervisor of intern training but if you are concerned about confidentiality you may feel more comfortable talking to your GP or seeking help from the Doctors Health Advisory Service* (see also Section 4.7 regarding doctors health advisory services).

Less predictable stresses are bullying or harassment, including sexual harassment, or lack of support that some interns will encounter.[20] At last, these problems are being spoken about and written about, and hopefully acted upon, so that the environment for interns and other healthcare workers should become universally supportive. If you are unlucky enough

---

* Doctors in training have reported that their rosters can make fitting in medical or counselling appointments problematic. Your Doctors Health Advisory Service should be willing to talk to you by telephone in the first instance and will be able to guide you to counsellors and GPs who can see you outside your rostered hospital hours.

to work in a hospital unit that allows bullying or is dysfunctional in other ways, dealing with the experience will not be easy. You will undoubtedly feel that if you make a complaint, it may be placed on your record and may impede your job prospects for the following year. Who to turn to will not always be immediately clear, especially if you are working in a hospital that you don't yet know well. From my experience, I would suggest first speaking with your medical education officer and then the supervisor of intern training. If you are so distressed that these options seem difficult, you should first seek support and counselling external to the hospital and in most parts of Australia this will be through the state or territory Doctors Health Advisory Service. Alternatively, if you have a GP who is interested in the well-being of doctors, you should first seek that doctor's advice.

The nature of some of the stresses experienced will almost certainly change over the years of your training as a junior doctor, and change again when you are in independent practice. Stress may be greatest at times of transition, as we have seen for the transition from student to intern. More advanced trainees find themselves weighed down by paperwork, clinical targets such as the four hour rule for patients to be seen and processed in the Emergency Department, time limits for standard operations, and statistics on their own performance such as finalising discharge summaries.[21] Understanding where the stresses might come from, learning about your response to any stress and knowing when and how to seek support or professional help is important, not least in helping you choose your career path wisely (see below). It may be helpful to be aware that medical practice will nearly always bring stresses and to also be aware that responses to any particular source of stress vary considerably between doctors. Some of the approaches described in this book to help you through the medical student years and some of the education now provided in the medical course about personal and professional development should help you in coping with these phases of your career as a doctor.

Firth-Cozens has extensively researched the stresses of medical and hospital practice for doctors in the United Kingdom and much of what she has found is likely to apply in Australia.[22] She notes that in addition to the unavoidable stresses of caring for patients, there are other aspects of the job of being a doctor that you might find are stressful or which, in a less supportive environment, might make clinical stresses more difficult to cope with. She points out that organisations such as hospitals, and hospital departments, vary in their culture and style of management and an unhappy more stressful working environment may result. Within hospital departments, the leadership and approach taken towards teamwork can also strongly influence how individual doctors feel about workloads and stresses. A good team should demonstrate open communication, friendliness, trust, mutual support, and shared and agreed goals. In such teams, patient care is better and mistakes occur less often. In the UK, shortened working hours for junior doctors may have undermined the traditional sense of belonging to a team, with the sense of support and continuity that this offers, but to date this has not been an issue in Australia. As a medical student and intern you will almost certainly observe that some hospital departments and teams seem to be happier places in which to work than others.

Tyssen and colleagues in Norway have also undertaken long term studies of medical graduates, examining the balance between individual and institutional factors contributing to stress during internship.[23] They found that vulnerability personality trait,* perceived recording skills, numbers of hours of sleep when on call, and the learning environment on the hospital wards were predictors of job stress. They noted that the vulnerability trait was especially important for female interns. They concluded that approaches to the prevention of stress should address both personal and institutional factors. A Swedish study of factors contributing to exhaustion in interns similarly emphasised the value of providing a supportive work environment in preventing exhaustion.[24]

It has become fashionable to speak of the inbuilt resilience of young doctors and to examine whether there are means by which resilience can be enhanced.[25] Some of those who write on this topic seem to ignore the

---

* Vulnerability in this study was assessed by a detailed questionnaire that included questions for example about levels of sensitivity to criticism and to the opinion of other people. The authors closely linked this trait with the trait of neuroticism (see footnote page 18).

impact of the environment in which young doctors work. In my view, it is highly likely that some unhealthy work environments will eventually strain the most resilient young doctor. I would place more emphasis on improving the work environment and less on inherent resilience. Other commentators agree,[26] many pointing out that young doctors have already proven their resilience through completing the medical course. This is not to downplay the potential value of 'resilience training' as it most often takes the form of helping young doctors cope with the stresses they are under.[27] When provided, it also demonstrates the value that any hospital holds for its junior medical staff, through giving the staff time for this activity and providing group sessions as a safe venue for debriefing and for feeling supported.

There are also steps that you can personally take to reduce the risk of burnout and help you to survive the stresses of the intern year. These include making time for regular exercise,[28] getting sufficient sleep,[29] discussing your work experiences with your peers, and maintaining contact with family and friends. Another option might be to access a program of mindfulness training now provided by some medical schools and hospitals.[30] Should you find yourself using drugs or alcohol to cope with stress and burnout, you should seek professional help sooner than later. Hazardous drinking either as a medical student or new graduate predicts similar issues in your later career.[31]

In some hospitals, you may be able to avail yourself of a scheme of peer support where you will be given the chance to pair with a graduate one or two years ahead of you. That person is then accessible for the entire twelve months to be your guide, mentor and advisor. In a controlled evaluation of such a program, the recipients of peer support were very satisfied with the program, and reported that it helped them to cope with stress, feel more supported and get greater job satisfaction.[32] You should obtain similar levels of support from a good registrar but as most intern rotations are a maximum of ten weeks, such support may be evanescent.

During the clinical training years that follow internship, studying for specialist examinations, applying for new jobs, having to relocate for clinical rotations, shift work and heavy workloads can all add to stress levels and can frequently lead to conflict between the demands of clinical work and of home life.[33]

Much has been done in Australia to seek to improve the working conditions of interns and other junior doctors. This has included introduction of rosters with safe working hours (see the 2002 Australian Medical Association's National Code of Practice – Hours of Work, Shift Work and Rostering for Hospital Doctors),[34] strengthening orientation programs for new interns, appointing senior doctors as training supervisors and creating the position of a medical education officer (MEO) in most hospitals. Although the original job description of the MEO was focussed on educational programs, MEOs in many hospitals have evolved to becoming key support personnel for interns and postgraduate year 2 (PGY2) doctors.

The AMA has since conducted a five yearly audit of safe working hours. The most recent was in 2016 and the results were published in July 2017.[35] The audit includes responses from trainee doctors and their senior consultants. For trainees it was of concern that the number of interns working rosters that placed them at risk of fatigue had increased since the last audit in 2011. This audit is a valuable exercise and hopefully most if not all junior doctors will participate each time it is conducted.

Through factors including night shifts, overtime work, and rural rotations, the intern year can be more stressful for interns with children. When seeking a suitable hospital for your intern year, you should ask questions about how supportive any hospital is likely to be if you are in this category. Some hospitals are prepared to offer paired intern rosters for medical couples.

5.4 Can the stress of the intern year be harmful?

For some interns, the answer is a resounding 'Yes'. Stress and burnout predispose to anxiety and depression. In young people who are used to being high achievers, depression can be devastating, through a combination of a sense of failure and the stigma that mitigates against seeking help. Almost every year in Australia, there are heart-breaking reports of suicide in young doctors. Recently a successful senior doctor went public about his failed attempt at suicide as a young doctor twenty-five years ago in the hope that anyone facing his dilemma these days will ask for help.[36] If you take no other message from this book, please realise that if you are struggling as an intern, independent help and support is readily available.

Stress and burnout, the latter often triggered by sleep deprivation, excess workload and mistreatment by superiors, and exacerbated via a lack of positive role models, are strongly linked to a decline in empathy for patients that has been observed to develop during the intern year. Diminished empathy bring with it risks of medical errors and lesser standard of patient care; patients will be aware of your lack of empathy. Additionally, Elton has suggested that loss of empathy may be linked to the subconscious repression of the difficult emotions that most interns experience.[37]

There are other risks of the intern year, including motor car accidents secondary to fatigue and the use of alcohol or licit or illicit drugs to relieve anxiety and symptoms of stress.

5.5 Tips for making the intern year enjoyable and rewarding

Earlier segments have focussed on how to keep healthy and cope with the stresses of the intern year. There are additional ways to ensure that the year is rewarding and enjoyable. One important means of making your life easier is to treat all hospital staff with respect and not get 'carried away' with your new medical degree. The staff members with whom you will interact most frequently are the nursing staff. It is rare to encounter a nurse who does not want to work cooperatively with doctors but if you are yourself uncooperative and inclined to look down upon nurses and not respect their intellects, role and skills, you are headed for a miserable year. In addition, experienced nurses know much more about practical aspects of medicine than do interns and can be of enormous assistance to receptive interns.

Everyone you work alongside with in our hospitals is dedicated to the care of patients. This includes technical staff in the investigative and laboratory services, the staff who deliver meals and the orderlies who assist in transporting patients among many others. Even if you are bad at remembering names, a cheerful smile and hello will be rewarded in other ways. Supervisors who report on your progress are likely to ask senior nurses about your attitude and performance so this alone should motivate you to show respect for all staff.

You should also take note of the role models that you encounter, especially your supervising registrar and consultant. If you encounter a negative role model, you will not be in a position to influence that person's conduct but being alert to good and bad role models will help you as you gradually become a fully trained doctor.[38]

Looking back on my own career as a junior doctor, one regret that I have is that I did not take time to read widely from the outset. I now believe that if you can make time for that, it will help you to become a better doctor.[39] For this reason, in this edition, as in the first, I have added as an appendix a list of books that might interest you. They are all related in some way to becoming a doctor and to the practice of medicine and thus while they are unlikely to help you to pass your specialist exams, they may make you a better and more insightful doctor.

As already mentioned, caring for yourself by making time for regular exercise,[40] getting sufficient sleep,[41] discussing your work experiences with your peers, and maintaining contact with family and friends will also help you enjoy the year. Should you find yourself using drugs or alcohol to cope with stress and burnout, you should seek professional help.

5.6 What if I find that I am not enjoying my intern year?

Two Australian surveys reported that almost one in five interns indicated that if they were to start over again, they would not choose to become doctors.[42] Thus if you feel unhappy or uncertain about your future as a doctor you are not alone. Nevertheless far fewer than 20% of interns or new doctors further along their training path give up medicine and change to another career. If you are unhappy and not sure that you are suited to a life in medicine, it is critical that you seek advice and counselling. A commonly under-recognised cause of lack of enjoyment is depression which is treatable so this needs to be excluded. If you are now in specialist training, it could be that you have unwisely chosen a field that does not suit you – again something that may be remediable, even if your career plans are delayed a little.

If you are not enjoying the intern year, you might also be struggling to cope with the workload and the responsibilities. This is not unusual and does not automatically mean that you are unsuited to be a doctor. It is a difficult year for some graduates but if you seek help and guidance, you might be pleasantly surprised with the outcome. Interns who are seen to be struggling may need help with their time management and priority setting skills or with identification of ways to enhance resilience or with advice about improving their knowledge base. Lack of real interest in your patients and their illnesses might be more difficult to address.[43]

It is also possible that you have indeed chosen a career for which you are unsuited. If this is the case, changing careers can be an emotionally wrenching and difficult decision.[44] Reports show that this difficulty can lead to graduates remaining in medicine for several more unhappy years while struggling to come to a decision. If you sense that this is your situation, I strongly recommend that you read a book written by Caroline Elton.[45] She is a UK based occupational psychologist who has long experience in assisting young doctors like you. Somewhere in her book, you are likely to find an account of another young doctor with whom you can identify. The cases in her book are likely to help you begin to understand why you feel the way you do. If you do seek counselling, this ideally should be with a clinical psychologist or psychiatrist with expertise and interest in this specialised field. Such a person may be best identified by your Doctors Health Advisory Service or Doctors Health Program.

5.7 Life after the intern year: The careers available in the Australian health care system.

By the end of your medical course and intern year, you are likely to have developed a reasonable understanding of Australia's complex health care system. However if you are reading this book as a potential medical student, a medical student in the early years of your course or an international student, you may benefit from reading a brief description of the health care system (see Attachment B) and thus better appreciate the very wide range of jobs open to medical graduates.

Potential or new medical students may also be puzzled by some of the confusing terminology of the medical workforce. Have you wondered what a physician does? The answer is that 'it depends' – depends, that is, on how and where the word 'physician' is used. If you hear it used on an American TV show, it will usually mean the equivalent of medical practitioner or doctor in the Australian context. In Australia, the word physician is primarily used to distinguish a large group of specialist doctors from surgeons, the major distinguishing feature being that physicians are trained to look after patients with conditions that do not require surgical operations. In addition, in Australia, the medical profession in speaking of a physician will most often be speaking about a specialist physician, one usually trained under the aegis of the Royal Australasian College of Physicians (see below), and will not be speaking about a general medical practitioner. General medical practitioners or 'general practitioners' (GPs) are also at times called family medicine physicians or primary care physicians. To confuse you further, specialist physicians are also at times called consultant physicians, a term related to the fact that these physicians 'consult' upon patients referred to them by general practitioners, and do not accept patients without such referrals.

There also exists a confusing array of terminology for the various stages of postgraduate medical training which commences with the intern year and this is explained in Section 5.8 below.

5.8 When should I begin to think about the field of medicine that I want to pursue? What do I need to do after the intern year?

Many students around the world have asked that more information about career options be made available to them well before graduation. As a medical student undertaking various clinical placements, you will begin to think about your choice as you see some of what each area of medical practice entails and as you observe various role models. Most students tend to change their mind about career choice over time.[46] In Australia the intern year and the subsequent one or even two years after graduation offer general experience so there is no need to commit to a particular path before graduation.

When first contemplated, the pathway from intern to an independent general practitioner or other independent specialist may seem long, complex and difficult to take in. The Australian Medical Association's website contains an excellent flow-chart depicting this path that is well worthwhile looking at.[47]

If you have not already done so, during your intern year it will be necessary for you to focus your mind on your future career direction, initially at a fairly broad level, i.e. are you thinking of becoming a general/family practitioner or a specialist in another field? If you are thinking of becoming a specialist,* is this in an area of surgery or internal medicine (physician) or are you attracted to general practice or psychiatry or paediatrics or to one of the 'investigative' branches of medicine such as radiology or pathology? This will heavily influence the nature of the hospital position you will seek in your next two years after the intern year. Specialist training programs are conducted by the various colleges (e.g. the Royal Australasian College of Surgeons, the Royal Australasian College of Physicians and others as detailed below) and each college has slightly different requirements for the clinical experience they wish their applicants for training to have.

---

* Although it remains common to restrict the term 'specialist' to doctors who pursue a clinical career other than general practice, it should be noted that in Australia general practice is also regarded as a specialty, with training and AMC accreditation requirements equivalent to the other specialties.

The formal training programs of the various colleges usually commence after either two or three years of predominantly hospital-based employment. The second year* (PGY2) has much in common with the intern year. These first two or three years after graduation, also known as pre-vocational training, are intended to provide a grounding for subsequent vocational (specialist) training, with varying degrees of specialisation in the rotations offered (e.g. in PGY2, you can choose a stream from one of several including 'medical', 'surgical', 'critical care' – covering emergency medicine, intensive care and anaesthetics – and 'general' streams, or work in paediatric or obstetric hospitals). In all of these streams you will usually rotate through subspecialty units each 2–3 months. In some PGY2 posts, you may work alongside an intern and contribute to the intern's training.

Employing hospitals provide formal educational programs and employ medical education officers to coordinate these training programs. The PGY2 programs are usually subject to external accreditation by the state based postgraduate medical education councils.† These councils come together as the Confederation of Postgraduate Medical Education Councils (CPMEC). CPMEC has strived for commonality of the training experience across Australia. Like the intern year, PGY2 doctors are supervised and supported by registrars‡ and senior doctors (consultants)

---

* In addition to the terms intern (PGY1) and PGY2, there is a profusion of terminology used in different states covering the first three years of postgraduate training. For example in Queensland, the PGY2 and PGY3 years are known as Junior House Officer and Senior House Officer respectively. In NSW, Resident Medical Officer is still used although residency in the hospital was done away with decades ago. In Victoria, the term Hospital Medical Officer years 1, 2 and 3, (with year 1 being the intern year) are used.

† The postgraduate medical education council in NSW is called the Health Education and Training Institute.

‡ A registrar is the name given to a doctor in training who is given additional responsibilities, usually after completion of PG years 1 to 3. Other than in general practice, the position of registrar nearly always involves the oversight and support of interns and other doctors in years PGY2 and 3. Most registrar positions are also accredited by a particular medical college and the registrar will be a trainee of that college and will be preparing for the examinations of the college. The number of years spent as a registrar before becoming qualified for independent

but are generally expected to take more responsibility than an intern. This period of prevocational training helps young doctors decide what specialty they might wish to pursue and at the same time brings valuable clinical learning opportunities and new skills. Each year usually brings an increased level of responsibility. In PGY3, rotations among various clinical units is the norm, although sometimes the rotations may be longer and in some positions, there may be the additional responsibility of supervising an intern.

Most medical graduates make a decision to enter a specialist (including general practice) training program in PGY2, PGY3 or PGY4. While the choice at this point may seem final, this is not so as some doctors change career direction during or after completion of their general practice or other specialist training. These training programs are provided by the medical colleges. The colleges accredit positions in health services, hospitals and general practice, provide teaching programs and conduct examinations for admission to fellowship. Detailed information is available on each college website (see Table 2 on page 117). If you are thinking of applying for a general practice registrar (training) position, you should seek advice about what hospital rotations may be accepted as contributing to the training time for general practice. Advice can be obtained from Australian General Practice Training.[48] During both PGY2 and PGY3 years, but especially the latter, most doctors begin to apply themselves to additional theoretical and clinical study in preparation for the written and clinical examinations involved for their chosen future area of practice. This study has to be accommodated within a full-time hospital service position.

In recent years two new closely related position titles have evolved for hospital doctors. One is the career medical officer (CMO) and the other is the 'hospitalist'.[49] A CMO is a doctor employed full time by a hospital in a role that has responsibilities akin to those of a senior registrar but the

practice in family medicine or specialist practice is a minimum of three but may be longer according to the requirements of each medical college. Registrars usually assume increasing levels of responsibility and when advanced in their training may be authorised to undertake a range of surgical or other procedures without supervision.

doctor has chosen not to pursue specialist training with one of the medical colleges. The role has arisen to fill the service needs of hospitals and is often filled by international medical graduates who have been unable to complete the requirements to have their prior specialist training recognised or upgraded in Australia. The position of the hospitalist was created in the USA and is a doctor whose only role is the care of hospital inpatients. Its relevance to Australian medicine is still uncertain.[50]

5.9 How much more training/time/exams are required after I graduate?

It is theoretically possible to commence independent medical practice immediately after the intern year. However, this is not advised for a number of reasons. From an ethical viewpoint, it is highly unlikely that your training and experience at that point would equip you adequately to provide even a reasonable standard of care for patients. In addition, you would not be entitled to receive Medicare rebates and either you or your patients would be financially disadvantaged. So despite this theoretical possibility, all Australian doctors who plan to enter independent medical practice undertake quite lengthy postgraduate study and training and complete the necessary assessments and examinations before entering practice.

The minimum time after graduation required to meet all the requirements for independent practice is about six years, although most specialists other than GPs take longer.[51] While these years involve study and sitting examinations, they also involve the clinical care of patients and during these years you will be earning an adequate salary. More information about post-graduate training pathways and their duration is found below.

5.10 Where can I get information and advice about careers for people with medical degrees?

During your time as a medical student and as an intern you will gradually be acquiring knowledge of many of the career options open to medical graduates and you will learn where to turn to for more information, advice and guidance. Each teaching hospital has a medical education officer and identified senior medical staff member(s) who can be approached for advice and information. In addition, in your clinical rotations as a student and as an intern, you will have the opportunity to observe at first-hand what is involved in many areas of medical practice. What follows is a summary of careers in medical practice.

The practice of clinical medicine in Australia is broadly divided between general /family medicine and the other specialty fields. The largest specialty fields, excluding general practice, are medicine and surgery and these fields may then be further subdivided into subspecialties. Used in this career context, 'medicine' generally refers to internal medicine and its sub-branches so as to distinguish it from the practice of surgery. Specialty fields in clinical medicine also include anaesthetics, obstetrics and gynaecology, psychiatry and paediatrics (including paediatric medicine, surgery and psychiatry). Newer specialties include pain medicine, palliative care medicine, addiction medicine, sexual health medicine and sports and exercise medicine. Although not usually involving direct clinical contact with patients, the health care system also needs doctors to practise in medical administration as well as in pathology (with its sub-branches of anatomical pathology, microbiology, biochemistry, immunology and haematology), radiology and medical imaging, including nuclear medicine.

In addition to choosing a career path in clinical medicine, laboratory or investigative medicine, medical administration and other fields, you will eventually also need to decide whether you wish to work in private practice, in the public health care system or a mixture of both.

You might also want to explore some less common career paths and employment opportunities for medical graduates. Some of these will involve you in clinical work to a greater or lesser degree, in fields such as academic medicine, forensic medicine, armed forces medicine and aviation medicine. Other fields such as administration (hospital, government department etc.), research, education, the pharmaceutical industry, the media and/or journalism, and business and management more generally, will take you away from patient contact.

A helpful website has been developed by the NSW Health Department to aid medical students and new graduates plan their careers and I strongly recommend it.[52] It not only describes each area of medical practice but also gives an indication as to whether any area is oversubscribed, undersubscribed or balanced in terms of popularity. There you may find attractive career options that you were unaware of or have not yet encountered.

The publication of the Australian Medical Association, the *Medical Journal of Australia*, includes a 'careers' segment in each fortnightly issue of the journal where most career opportunities are covered.*

5.11 Is there anything I should know about how or why medical graduates choose their careers?

The approach to choosing a long-term career has traditionally depended upon individuals simply trying to work out for themselves what they might do and how they might go about this. Usually one or more mentors were approached for guidance and support but how this happened depended upon the initiative of each trainee and the approachability of any mentor. This is gradually changing and becoming more formalised. In most states, each year a one day 'medical careers expo' is held, providing medical students and graduates with an opportunity to talk to representatives of the medical colleges and the teaching hospitals about career opportunities. Hospitals and colleges also hold 'career nights' where your questions can be answered. In the teaching hospitals, directors of training for the various

---

* Most of the advice is 'open access' and past contributions can be found at https://www.mja.com.au/search?search=careers.

programs (medicine, surgery, emergency medicine and so on) and medical education officers are available to discuss career options.

It may be difficult to obtain career advice about general practice via teaching hospitals. Alternative sources of advice and guidance include talking with your local GP, keeping in touch with any GPs you have encountered during your student rotations and talking with representatives of the GP training programs and colleges at a career's expo. The Royal Australian College of General Practitioners has an online General Practice Career Guide that you may find helpful.[53]

When asked what influenced their career choice, doctors commonly respond in terms of having enjoyed the clinical content of an area as a student or trainee and having been influenced positively by supportive and enthusiastic role models – registrars and senior doctors[54] and also negatively influenced by poor role models. Other factors include the nature of the work, the working hours (lifestyle/work-life balance),[55] diversity of the work,[56] career opportunity,[57] self-appraisal of skills, remuneration, and requirements for being on call after hours.[58] US studies indicate that factors such as controllable lifestyle, future income and educational debt influence career choice. From the UK, Elton has described the three key influences on career choice as the effect of role models, exposure to the type of work involved and work-life balance. She points out that there is a risk that a negative role model might deter you from a field that could otherwise be suitable.[59] An Australian survey indicated that only 16% of specialist trainees rated financial prospects as an important factor in career choice[60] but nevertheless the most keenly sought after positions are often the best paid. Male doctors appear more influenced by prestige and income while female doctors are more influenced by antisocial hours.[61] Some doctors do not enjoy continuity in caring for patients and choose careers with more variety (e.g. with components of research or teaching or some administration, or with patient contact not involving continuity of care such as radiology, anaesthetics or emergency medicine).

A major study of factors influencing choice of specialty including general practice commissioned by the Australian Medical Workforce

Advisory Committee obtained responses from 54% of 7,851 doctors in training in 2002.[62] The study reported that 'appraisal of own skills and aptitudes' (79% of respondents) and 'intellectual content of the specialty' (75%) were important factors, followed by 'work culture' (72%), 'flexibility of working arrangements' (56%) and 'hours of work' (54%). In this study, 80% of those surveyed had chosen their career by the end of the third year after graduation.

Research from the UK has shown that graduates who felt the most stress as interns tend to select careers with less stress, usually involving less direct patient care and/or less continuity of care, such as laboratory medicine, public health, medical imaging or anaesthetics. Follow-up assessments have suggested that these were wise decisions as the stress levels of doctors in these fields were reduced as compared to their stress levels as interns. A very notable exception was psychiatry where, on average, stress levels were quite high as interns but were even higher when these doctors entered psychiatric practice. It is suggested that their choice of psychiatry may have related to seeking to better understand themselves. This study showed that the least stressed group, both as students and when postgraduate training had been completed, were those who chose a career as surgeons. Collectively, this research suggests that much of the stress of medicine is related to the nature of any patient contact and that the experience of stress is influenced by factors personal to each doctor.[63]

A new non-rational influence on career choice has been a subject of interest, viz. what is called a basic emotional response of avoiding things that might be disgusting (also called 'disgust sensitivity'). Thus it has been proposed that this could be a factor discouraging women from choosing a career in surgery.[64]

You may also wish to reflect on other personal choices such as whether you enjoy doing procedures more than talking with patients (or vice versa) and whether you need variety or intellectual challenges to remain energetic and enthused about your work. In my own case, I found direct patient contact the most rewarding element of medical practice but also the most demanding. I marvelled at colleagues whose only work was patient care and who never wavered in their commitment, whereas I needed regular breaks, whether these came via research, teaching, administration or other interests, such as writing. Some of the influences on your career choice may not be conscious and if so, it may be that later you will find those very reasons are also the reasons why the area that you chose is unduly stressful.

The research group conducting the long term study of Australian doctors (the MABEL study referred to earlier)[65] has completed a 'stated preference discrete-choice experiment' aimed at better understanding what factors might influence career choices of doctors.[66] Several factors were identified including work-life balance (especially on call duties), the intrinsic attributes of any career, opportunities for procedural work, and educational debt. The authors suggested that the then trend away from choosing general practice could be reversed by adjusting incomes to be closer to those of specialists and providing more opportunity for procedural work for general practitioners.

Other factors that may need to be considered in choosing a career path include the needs of your family, your personality (it is claimed that GPs have to be able to cope with greater uncertainty than other doctors and that surgeons as a group seek a rapid sense of achievement in their work) and your working style (e.g. a need for independence as compared with working in a large organisation or in a team). The medical school you attended may also influence your career choice as some medical schools seek to foster a positive attitude to research while others may emphasise service to rural, remote, Indigenous or less privileged communities.

As mentioned earlier, with the growth in the number of medical graduates, there may be increased difficulty in obtaining your first choice of post graduate training in the more popular specialties. The limitations on the number of accredited training posts in some specialties, most notably surgery, have created additional dilemmas. In surgery, hospitals may offer employment in both accredited and 'non-accredited' registrar posts. In taking up a non-accredited post, your career is on hold as you wait and hope that eventually you will be offered an accredited spot. Some commentators worry that occupants of such posts and even those who are secure in an accredited post may feel pressured to work longer hours, mostly unpaid, to impress their supervisors and thus secure their career.[67] This is yet another matter to take into consideration in choosing your career direction.

Although there are now more female medical graduates than men, women remain under-represented in many areas of practice, especially in certain specialist fields. More time and effort may be needed to find supportive mentors and role models for areas of practice which women are considering. The general practice training program provides opportunities for part time training but this is more difficult in some types of hospital-based specialist training. A key issue for all young doctors, especially female doctors, will be seeking to balance work, family and lifestyle in any career choice.[68] It may well be that for junior doctors, work-life balance is more readily achieved through choosing a rural placement.[69]

UK-based occupational psychologist, Caroline Elton, has written an excellent book that is very relevant to career choices.[70] It covers a large range of issues, too many to summarise here. Several of the distressed doctors who sought her help with career advice were those who may have chosen their career because of unresolved and subconscious issues derived from their life before medical school, including the premature death of a parent or sibling or the presence of mental illness in the family. Her long experience leads her to advise that you should choose your area of practice with 'eyes wide open', noting that 'choosing one's specialty is a complex psychological decision'. If you are struggling with the matter of choice of specialty, and even if you are not, I commend her book to you.

5.12 Should interns take a close interest in information provided about medical workforce trends in Australia?

Planning for the medical workforce in Australia has a chequered history. Currently we are in a phase of expansion of the number of medical schools and medical graduates together with moves to reduce our intake of doctors trained in other countries.[71] This expansion, especially of medical graduates, is likely to increase competition for vocational training positions and via that competition place even more stress on trainees.

We are also in a phase where governments have taken steps to seek to entice more medical graduates to work in rural and remote medical practice, not only as GPs but also as medical, surgical and other specialists. As a medical student or new medical graduate, it is unlikely that careful study of government reports on workforce planning and workforce trends will be of much assistance to you.[72] While Australia's population continues to grow, so too will the need for doctors. A much more relevant workforce issue for young doctors is which areas of medical practice are undersubscribed or oversubscribed and the new NSW website mentioned earlier is likely to prove very helpful to you.

5.13 Tell me more about the medical colleges

The oversight of training in general practice/family medicine and all medical, surgical and other specialties is delegated in Australia to the medical colleges. The training program for general practitioners is coordinated by the Australian General Practice Training, with the training being provided predominantly by fellows of the Royal Australian College of General Practitioners and the Australian College of Rural and Remote Medicine. There are 16 medical colleges accredited by the Australian Medical Council to provide vocational specialty training (see Table 3 below). Colleges historically were established by groups of doctors with similar interests in order that the training of future doctors in that field could be assured and that the continuing education needs of the group could be supported. The largest Australian college in terms of its membership is the Royal Australian College of General Practitioners. The oldest is the Royal Australasian College of Surgeons which was founded in 1931. Prior to that time, Australian specialists sought membership of UK colleges. The other colleges cover internal medicine (physicians), obstetrics and gynaecology, anaesthetics, pathology, radiology, psychiatry, dermatology, emergency medicine, ophthalmology, sports medicine and medical administration. Nearly all of these colleges serve both Australia and New Zealand, explaining why many use the title 'Australasian'.

Table 3: The Australian medical colleges accredited by the Australian Medical Council

(See also https://www.amc.org.au/accreditation-and-recognition/ assessment-accreditation-specialist-medical-programs-assessment- accreditation-specialist-medical-programs/specialist-medical-colleges/)

Australasian College of Sport and Exercise Physicians (ACSEP)	www.acsep.org.au
Australasian College for Emergency Medicine (ACEM)	www.acem.org.au
Australian College of Rural and Remote Medicine (ACRRM)	www.acrrm.org.au
Australasian College of Dermatologists (ACD)	www.dermcoll.edu.au
Australian and New Zealand College of Anaesthetists (ANZCA)	www.anzca.edu.au
Faculty of Pain Medicine (FPM)	www.fpm.anzca.edu.au
College of Intensive Care Medicine of Australia and New Zealand (CICM)	www.cicm.org.au
Royal Australasian College of Dental Surgeons (RACDS)	www.racds.org
Royal Australian College of General Practitioners (RACGP)	www.racgp.org.au
Royal Australasian College of Medical Administrators (RACMA)	www.racma.edu.au
Royal Australasian College of Physicians (RACP)*	www.racp.edu.au

---

* The RACP includes the Adult Medicine Division, the Paediatrics and Child Health Division, the Australasian Faculty of Rehabilitation Medicine, the Australasian Faculty of Occupational and Environmental Medicine, the Australasian Faculty of Public Health Medicine, the Australasian Chapter of Palliative Medicine, the Australian Chapter of Addiction Medicine and the Australasian Chapter of Sexual Health Medicine.

Royal Australasian College of Surgeons (RACS)	www.surgeons.org
Royal Australian and New Zealand College of Ophthalmologists (RANZCO)	www.ranzco.edu
Royal Australian and New Zealand College of Obstetricians and Gynaecologists (RANZCOG)	www.ranzcog.edu.au
Royal Australian and New Zealand College of Psychiatrists (RANZCP)	www.ranzcp.org
Royal Australian and New Zealand College of Radiologists (RANZCR)	www.ranzcr.edu.au
Royal College of Pathologists of Australasia (RCPA)	www.rcpa.edu.au

In addition to the accredited colleges, there are some other organisations that are not accredited by the Australian Medical Council but also call themselves colleges. Some of these provide support for clinical training and provide continuing medical education for their members, and may eventually seek accreditation by the Australian Medical Council (e.g. the Australian College of Cosmetic Surgery) while others are more akin to a special interest association or society (e.g. the Australian College of Legal Medicine).

Entry to training programs of many of the colleges is very competitive. So too can be the pursuit of preferred hospital or family medicine training positions. The processes for selection into training programs and hospital and general practice training positions vary considerably and are likely to be modified.[73] While many of the colleges divide their training program into basic and advanced training, there is considerable variation in the content and requirements of the programs. Much of the study involved in preparing for college examinations is self-directed. However, colleges are increasingly providing detailed curricula and formal teaching programs. There are fees for joining a college training program and for their examinations, and the pass* rates for the colleges' examinations are generally lower than pass rates

---

* Pass rates may change as the previous approach of some colleges to use examinations to rank trainees for entry into the next phase of training is replaced by 'criterion referenced' examination standards as required for AMC accreditation.

at medical school. However, the vast majority of those who embark on postgraduate training eventually complete that training. This phase of the medical career brings its own particular stresses.

The training programs of the medical colleges are demanding for junior doctors; finding time to study for the theoretical and clinical examinations conducted by the colleges while gaining hands on clinical experience in hospital or family practice, carrying a service workload, supervising interns, and meeting family or personal commitments can be very challenging. The time taken from graduation from medical school to completion of postgraduate training as a specialist and finding a hospital appointment can be as long as nine years. This time will be extended if you include research training (e.g. towards another degree such as a PhD) and/or some further clinical or research training overseas. The time to complete vocational training for general practice is on average six years after graduation.

In addition to providing training programs and conducting fellowship examinations, the medical colleges provide for the continuing education of their fellows and develop professional and ethical standards for their fellows. Most also provide information on health matters to the general community.

Within many colleges, there is provision for subspecialisation. For example, the Royal Australasian College of Physicians (RACP) has adult medicine and paediatric medicine divisions as well as additional 'faculties' and 'chapters' covering public health physicians and physicians in rehabilitation medicine, occupational medicine, addiction medicine and sexual health medicine. Fellows of the adult medicine and paediatric medicine divisions of the RACP can opt to specialise in a wide range of fields including allergy, cardiology, endocrinology, gastroenterology, geriatrics, haematology, hepatology, hypertension, immunology, infectious diseases, oncology, nephrology, neurology, pharmacology, rheumatology or respiratory medicine. RACP fellows can also practice as generalists in internal medicine and cover all these areas, but not to the same depth as a subspecialist.

Similar sub-specialisation occurs in surgery and to a lesser degree in other areas of medical practice. For example, fellows of the RACS may choose to be general surgeons or specialise in such fields as cardiac surgery, neurosurgery, orthopaedics, vascular surgery, upper gastrointestinal surgery, colorectal surgery, thoracic surgery, and ear nose and throat surgery. In paediatric internal medicine and in paediatric surgery, a similar range of specialist and subspecialist fields apply. However, training in and subsequent practice of paediatric specialist medicine or surgery is confined to children and it is now quite rare for anyone other than a general practitioner to conduct a practice that involves caring for both adults and children. In addition, although much more informal in their development and training, 'special interests' such as in acupuncture or hypnotherapy may be pursued and practised by general practitioners and other specialists.

Making a decision about the field of medicine in which you will practise is as important as the decision you faced when you first read this book and decided to enrol at medical school. The more time you put into thinking about the role for which you might be most suited and researching your options and what each entails, the more likely it is that you will be happy with your decision. Fortunately, choosing an area of medicine to train for and practise in is not a decision that has to be made quickly. During your clinical rotations as a medical student and during your intern year and second year of clinical experience, you will have ample opportunity to observe many areas of medical practice and discuss with teachers and mentors why they chose the area they are in and seek their advice. In these discussions, you will also often hear that many doctors do change career direction at various points in their lives and will be reassured that no decision about any career in medicine has to be regarded as permanent.

Attachment A: The Medical Board of Australia, the regulation of the medical profession and the governance of the health care system

The medical profession is described as 'self-regulating' and this remains partly true in Australia. To practise medicine in Australia, one needs to be registered with the Medical Board of Australia (MBA), a body established under a 'national' law. The majority of members of the MBA are themselves medical practitioners, as are the majority of members of state-based branches of the MBA. The MBA registers appropriately qualified persons, meaning graduates of a medical school accredited by the AMC and international medical graduates who have been individually assessed by the AMC. In addition to the task of registering medical practitioners, the other roles of the MBA, consistent with its primary purpose of protecting the public, include developing and issuing guidelines as to the standards expected of doctors (e.g. the MBA *Code of Good Medical Practice* as referred to in Section 1.1), handling complaints made about doctors and assessing doctors who through ill health may be impaired and temporarily or permanently not able to practise medicine safely. Most of these matters are dealt with by the state and territory branches of the MBA. In all of these tasks, the MBA works with or is supported by the AHPRA. Where complaints raise possible issues of misconduct (see endnote), these are investigated by AHPRA with the MBA state branch and if deemed serious will be referred to a disciplinary hearing. The process for disciplinary hearings varies between states and territories but allegations of serious misconduct are assessed by a panel or tribunal usually consisting of a senior lawyer and two experienced medical practitioners.

Under the national law, medical schools are obliged to have medical students registered with the MBA. The powers of the MBA in regard to medical students are confined to matters relating to student health and student behaviour that could place patients at risk. Registration of students is free. The process of registration means that medical students should regularly receive communications from the MBA and thus, well before graduation, made aware of its role and its expectations of doctors.

After graduation, new doctors must undertake a year of supervised practice (the intern year) and for this year, registration with the MBA is 'provisional'. To be provisionally registered the new graduate must meet English language standards, provide proof of identity, provide evidence of medical indemnity insurance and complete a criminal history check. At the completion of the intern year and provided that performance has been satisfactory, the MBA grants full registration. Assessment of intern performance is based on reports received from intern supervisors at the end of each rotation. Each hospital has to submit a statement to the MBA attesting to the fact that progress has been satisfactory and recommending that the intern should be granted full registration. Once a doctor has full registration, in theory, he or she is legally permitted to practise without supervision. However, almost all junior doctors continue to train and gain experience under gradually diminishing levels of supervision for a number of years, for reasons including restricted access to Medicare payments for doctors without post graduate general practice or specialist qualifications.

In addition to the process of medical registration and the powers of the Medical Board of Australia in relation to alleged misconduct and impairment, there are legal and other controls and constraints on the practice of medicine. While these controls and constraints are of little daily consequence to most doctors in how they practise in their chosen field, medical students will gradually be made aware of them. In no particular order, they include some formal and informal controls over the scope of medical practice, primarily relating to training and qualifications. For example public and private hospitals will only employ or give a right of practice in any particular field to doctors who are appropriately qualified and trained for the particular role. Other 'controls' include the existence of health complaints commissioners in every state, the right of patients to sue for negligence, the legislation surrounding Medicare (covering over-servicing and fraud) and state-based legislation in regard to storing, prescribing and administering drugs of addiction.

Medical knowledge continues to grow and medical practice is constantly changing. Maintenance of professional standards and competence throughout a doctor's working life is expected by the community and most doctors pursue continuing education as a matter of both habit and enjoyment. Doctors are supported in this via the educational activities and programs of medical colleges and other professional societies. When renewing their medical registration each year with the MBA, doctors must provide evidence of their participation in a continuing education program.

Endnote

The Health Practitioner Regulation National Law Act 2009 defines notifiable conduct (i.e. possible misconduct that warrants investigation and could lead to disciplinary action) as including: practising medicine while intoxicated by alcohol or drugs; engaging in sexual misconduct in connection with the practice of medicine; and placing the public at risk of harm because the doctor has practised medicine in a way that constitutes a significant departure from accepted professional standards. The legislation also defines unprofessional conduct as professional conduct that is of a lesser standard than that which might be expected of the health practitioner by the public or the practitioner's professional peers and goes on to list a number of specific examples.

Attachment B: The Australian health care system – a brief description

The Australian health care system is a complex entity with many components.[74] One means of describing the system is to consider its 'public' and 'private' components. Most but not all the large hospitals in Australia are public hospitals funded by government and are accessible to all, usually at no cost to the patient. Most public hospitals are general hospitals, providing a full range of services but a small number are devoted only to single fields such as paediatrics, obstetrics and gynaecology, psychiatry, cancer or ophthalmology.

The medical staff of public hospitals include full-time and part-time senior doctors (the latter referred to most often as visiting medical officers or VMOs) and large numbers of junior doctors in various stages of training (with the titles of interns, 'residents' or hospital medical officers, and registrars). These hospitals are usually also identified as 'teaching' hospitals because they provide clinical experience and teaching to medical students as well as providing most specialist medical training, other than the training of general (family medicine) practitioners. Each teaching hospital is usually affiliated with one university medical school although a few hospitals take students from more than one medical school. Senior doctors often hold both hospital and academic (medical school/university) appointments. These doctors play a large role in teaching medical students and in supervising and teaching junior doctors. Most universities have established university departments (e.g. departments of medicine and of surgery) and 'clinical schools' within their affiliate hospitals to foster clinical teaching and research. The clinical school will be the 'home base' for medical students allocated to that hospital. A very small number of teaching hospitals in Australia are conducted as 'university' hospitals, where the state government (responsible for public hospitals) facilitates the integration of the academic teaching staff into the management of the hospital. Teaching hospitals also play an important part in training nursing graduates, allied health professionals, medical scientists and most of the other disciplines and trades required by hospitals and the health care system.

There is also a well-developed sector of private hospitals, large and small, some of which are conducted as not-for-profit institutions by religious organisations. Patients are admitted to private hospitals under the care of individual specialists who have sole medical responsibility for the patient's care. Patients are billed for all services although in practice most of the bills are met via a combination of the patient's private health insurance and Medicare (see below). Most private hospitals do not have junior doctors on staff and many do not provide training for medical students but this is gradually changing. Most private hospitals do not provide an emergency department and not all have intensive care units. As a result the range of illnesses and injuries treated in these hospitals is narrower than in the public hospitals.

Another distinction between public and private hospitals is that in general most medical research in Australia that involves patients has historically been conducted in the public hospital sector, but research is gradually expanding into the private sector.

As well as there being a public/private divide among hospitals, there is also a divide in the care of patients who do not need hospital care (the vast majority). In general medical practice, the public/private divide is somewhat obscured by the funding system. Most general practice is part of the private system so that if a person seeks medical care from a general practitioner, that person is responsible for meeting any costs involved. The costs of care in general practice, and for attending a private specialist, are defrayed or in many instances completely reimbursed by the national health insurance scheme known as Medicare (see below re 'bulk billing' and Medicare). Most general practitioners are self-employed (i.e. are not employees of government or part of the public service). Some general practice services in some states are provided by community health services established by government, usually in economically less well-off areas. The general practitioners in these services may be employees of the service or may have a 'fee for service' contract. These clinics are attractive to some doctors as they usually provide an onsite comprehensive service, employing dieticians, physiotherapists, counsellors and other health professionals.

Specialist surgical and medical care, including mental health care, is available both through the private system and via the public hospital system. The majority of specialist doctors work in both the public and private systems. In private practice, many specialists work in individual practices, although some share office space, overheads and staff with colleagues and a proportion have formal systems of sharing on-call after hours cover. Access to specialist care requires a referral from a general practitioner. Without a referral, the patient is not entitled to claim a rebate of the cost of care from Medicare. This referral pathway also ensures that the patient's general practitioner is the overall coordinator of care and the central record keeper for the patient.

Although Australia has one of the world's most equitable health care systems, Medicare rebates have not kept pace with the fees charged in both general and specialist medical practice. In general practice, over 70% of consultations are 'bulk-billed' so that the majority of patients do not have to meet out of pocket expenses. In specialist practice, bulk-billing rates are much lower, although many specialists bulk bill (or accept the Medicare rebate as full payment) if the patient is a pensioner or has a chronic illness requiring repeated attendances. It is illegal for private health care funds to offer insurance to meet any out of pocket charges, other than when a patient is admitted to hospital for investigation or treatment. When a patient is admitted privately, the combination of reimbursements from Medicare and from a private health fund ensures that many patients do not have out of pocket expenses.

Most public teaching hospitals provide a full range of specialist outpatient clinics where patients are seen at no charge. These clinics are staffed by part-time (VMOs) and/or full-time specialists together with junior doctors in training. For junior doctors, as well as for medical students, these clinics provide opportunities to see and learn from patients with a wide range of problems and illnesses that do not require inpatient admission. Through access to new and/or experimental treatments and new investigative techniques, public hospital outpatient clinics provide access to care, sometimes long term, for patients with complex or uncommon conditions, care that may not be available in the private system.

There is considerable movement of patients, doctors and information between the private and public health care systems. Patients are often referred by general practitioners to public hospitals for specialist consultations, investigation and inpatient care. Specialists in private practice are keen to maintain links with at least one public hospital and thus seek appointment as VMOs. One of the attractions of these appointments is that they provide teaching contact with medical students. In addition inpatients are frequently transferred between public and private hospitals. Transfer to a public hospital might occur when severity of illness, need for access to technology or particular levels of care, or adequacy of health insurance is at issue. Transfer out of a public hospital to a private hospital might be requested by a patient wanting more privacy (e.g. a single room).

Another way of explaining the health care system is to examine the divide between primary medical care and specialist medical care. For people who are unwell and wish to see a doctor, most primary medical care is provided by general (family) medical practitioners who are self-employed in that part of the health care system described as private. However, some primary care is provided via community health centres where the doctors are likely to be employees. In addition, seriously ill persons, and even some who are less seriously ill, may go straight to a hospital emergency department for medical attention. While nearly all emergency departments are based within large public hospitals, a small but increasing number can be found in private hospitals.

A growing trend in Australia is the establishment of 'corporate' general practice, as well as corporatisation of radiology and pathology. Business entities, some owned by doctors, purchase existing medical practices or build new practices and staff the practices entirely with general practitioners (or radiologists or pathologists as the case may be) who may be independent contractors or salaried employees. The attraction for the owners is profit while for the employee doctors the attractions include avoiding the work of managing and hiring staff and running the business, as well as opportunities to work part-time. Critics of this trend allege that poorer standards of care and lack of continuity of care can follow.

In urban areas, it is often stated that GPs have been deskilled in recent years. A number of procedural areas of clinical practice including obstetrics, surgery, anaesthetics, and managing trauma are no longer the domain of urban GPs. It is now very unusual that GPs in urban areas will arrange, or are even permitted to arrange, to admit a patient to a private or public hospital under their own care. However, the length, quality and complexity of the training available to GPs has increased and skills in other areas, including counselling and preventive medicine, have been strengthened.

Over time, the work of GPs in remote and rural areas of Australia has diverged significantly from their urban colleagues. Doctors in remote and rural areas are required to provide a wider range of procedural aspects of clinical practice than do their urban colleagues. This has resulted in the establishment of a second 'GP' college, the Australian College of Rural and Remote Medicine, to meet the training and continuing education needs of this group of doctors as well as the provision of additional rural general practice training by the Royal Australian College of General Practitioners.

APPENDICES

1. Additional relevant websites

(The websites of the Australian medical schools can be found on pages 57–75 and the websites of the Australian medical colleges can be found on pages 139–40.)

Australian Council on Educational Research www.acer.edu.au

Australian General Practice Training www.agpt.com.au

Australian Indigenous Doctors' Association www.aida.org.au

Australian Medical Association www.ama.com.au

Australian Medical Council www.amc.org.au

Australian Medical Students Association www.amsa.org.au

Australian Medical Students Journal www.amsj.org

Confederation of Postgraduate Medical Education Councils www.cpmec.org.au

Graduate Australian Medical School Admissions Test (GAMSAT) www.gamsat.acer.edu.au

Medical Board of Australia www.medicalboard.gov.au

Medical Deans Australia and New Zealand www.medicaldeans.org.au

University Clinical Aptitude Test www.ucat.edu.au

2. Suggested further reading

Unseen. The secret world of a chronic illness. Parsons J. Affirm Press, South Melbourne, Victoria, 2020. If you only read one book from this list, this should be it. Jacinta Parsons is a Melbourne journalist and radio presenter who has suffered from Crohn's disease since she was a university student. This account of her experiences will open your eyes to aspects of illness and patient care that are often ignored. It will allow you to see the health care system through the eyes of the patient, encourage you to truly listen to the patient's story and help you to understand why the science of medicine must be combined with the humanity.

How to Succeed at Medical School: An Essential Guide to Learning. Evans D and Brown J. Wiley-Blackwell BMJ Books, UK, 2009. This short book looks at both the theory and practice of the learning involved at medical school. It is written by two UK academic teachers with considerable experience in helping medical students to learn. It contains a large amount of very clear practical advice for all stages of the medical course as well as advice about revision and tackling examinations.

How Doctors Think: Clinical Judgement and the Practice of Medicine. Montgomery K. Oxford University Press, New York, 2006. This is a very well written and researched book from an American academic with a background in ethics and humanities who has worked closely with doctors in hospitals and has critically analysed the 'science' of medicine. To quote from the introduction: 'In undertaking the care of a patient, physicians – however scientific they may be – are not engaged in a quantifiable science but in a rational interpretive practice.' In addition she was drawn in to observing and commenting on the hierarchical staff relationships she found.

How Doctors Think. Groopman J. Scribe Publications, Carlton North, Victoria, 2007. Also written about American medicine, this 'US best seller' is a very different book to that of Dr Montgomery. Dr Groopman approaches his theme with accounts of how other doctors (those who he clearly holds in high esteem) successfully think and work their way through a variety of challenging clinical problems. Each story contains many lessons for doctors, both new and more experienced.

This Going to Hurt: Secret Diaries of a Junior Doctor. Adam Kay. Picador, London, 2017. This book is likely to be most enjoyable if read several months in to your intern year. Written by a UK doctor who graduated in 2004 and worked in British National Health Service hospitals for the next six years, this book is funny and insightful, at times disrespectful, and eventually quite sad.

Tiger's Eye: A Memoir. Clendinnen I. Text Publishing, Melbourne, Victoria, 2000. While much of this wonderfully written memoir by an acclaimed Australian writer has little to do with medicine and hospitals, it also contains some searing and vivid descriptions of what it is really like to be seriously ill and an inpatient in modern Australian public hospitals. Without becoming ill yourself, this is as close as you might ever get to that reality.

Tell Me the Truth: Conversations with My Patients About Life and Death. Srivastava R. Viking Camberwell, Victoria, 2010. If you do not get to read this book before or during your student days, it is a must read after graduation. It is beautifully written account of how a young Australian doctor came to choose her specialty of oncology (cancer medicine) and about her 'learning curve' in the specialty. Among the many messages it contains, the most powerful are about the importance of listening to patients and respecting their individual stories and about the impact of role models (positive and negative) in medicine.

Dissection. Jacinta Halloran. Scribe Publications, Carlton North, Victoria, 2008. In reading this book, most doctors would rapidly forget this is fiction, so convincingly depicted is the central character, a Melbourne female general practitioner, whose life is upturned on being sued for a missed diagnosis of a bone cancer in a teenage boy. While the law suit underpins the story, there is much more to learn about the highs and lows of medical practice through reading this story, beautifully written by a practising doctor.

Breaking and Mending: A Junior Doctor's Stories of Compassion and Burnout. Joanna Cannon. Profile Books, London, 2019. The author left school at the age of 15 but returned to study medicine in her 30s, with a burning wish to become a psychiatrist. In this memoir she describes her struggles with aspects of her UK medical course and her intern year in the NHS. She also depicts insightfully her emotionally charged interactions with seriously ill patients and their families and reflects on the pressures that lead some young doctors to suicide.

The Doctor in Literature: Satisfaction or Resentment. Posen S. Radcliffe Publishing, Oxford, UK, 2005. This book is the first of a series written by Dr Solomon Posen, an Australian physician, which explores in depth how doctors have been portrayed in literature throughout history. He has used the literature to demonstrate that the general community's attitudes towards doctors and the failings of many fictional doctors have altered little over time. Each chapter concludes with short summaries that reflect not only what his research has found but also his own insights gained from a long career in clinical medicine. This is a book to be delved into from time to time as your career progresses.

GLOSSARY

burnout: a combination of emotional exhaustion, depersonalisation and/or reduced feelings of personal accomplishment that can occur in persons whose study or work commitments have been very demanding and/or stressful.

clinical practice: the work most commonly undertaken by doctors, usually involving consulting with patients, taking a history, conducting a physical examination, arranging tests, making a diagnosis and providing treatment.

clinical rotation: the practice of moving medical students and junior doctors through a series of medical, surgical and other specialty services. For junior doctors a rotation is usually of 10–14 weeks' duration.

compassion fatigue: the apparent lack of empathy and concern for patients and mechanistic approach to patients that can occur in doctors who are overworked, stressed or suffering burnout.

consortium: the group of graduate-entry medical schools that have collaborated in the development of GAMSAT, or the separate group of undergraduate-entry medical schools that have collaborated in the application of UCAT.

extraversion: a term used in psychology and the opposite of introversion. An extrovert will typically be outgoing and sociable while an introvert will be reserved and shy.

fellow: on completing a specialty training program and becoming a member of a medical college, a doctor is awarded the 'fellowship' of the college, hence the term fellow.

grade point average (GPA): a measure of academic performance used in university assessment where performance in each subject or unit is graded from pass (4), credit (5), distinction (6) and high distinction (7) or similar scale. The

GPA is the average grade achieved over the course of a degree. The GPA can be weighted to take account of more recent performance.

graduate entry (GE): a graduate-entry medical course is one where students cannot enrol without first completing another university degree.

intern/internship: the compulsory year of predominantly hospital-based practical experience, spent under supervision, which all medical graduates must complete before they can be granted full registration by the Medical Board of Australia.

junior doctor: a term applied to recent medical graduates, including interns, who are undertaking supervised postgraduate training. In the hospital setting, this is contrasted with senior doctors/senior medical staff who are authorised to practise independently.

medical college: the generic name given to the Australian medical organisations that are responsible for postgraduate training and assessment of specialists (including general practitioners) and for continuing education of the college fellowship.

medical practice: see clinical practice.

neuroticism: a basic personality trait described in psychology as an enduring tendency to experience negative emotional states. People who score highly for this trait are more likely to experience feelings of guilt, anxiety or depression and to respond less well to environmental stress.

postgraduate medical council: a state-based government-supported body responsible for the accreditation of training positions for doctors in the intern and second postgraduate year, and for the support and oversight of training of these doctors.

postgraduate training: the period spent in training, and gaining clinical experience under supervision, between graduation and becoming qualified for independent medical practice (see also pre-vocational and vocational training).

preventive medicine: in the context of general practice (family medicine) refers to steps taken to prevent illness (e.g. by immunisation) or to screen for illness at an early stage (e.g. breast cancer screening).

pre-vocational training: the time spent in the first two or three years of postgraduate training gaining general experience before commencing training in a dedicated area of medicine (the latter being known as vocational training – see below).

problem-based learning: there is no one agreed definition of problem-based learning but this learning method is likely to have the following features: students are required to work collaboratively in small groups; the problem (usually based around a clinical case) is explored in depth over a period of a week or two; and a trained tutor acts as facilitator, supporting the group in self-directed study to achieve the learning objectives of the current problem.

procedural work: a subsection of clinical practice whereby a patient undergoes some form of diagnostic or treatment 'procedure', e. g. minor or major surgery or other procedure such as endoscopy, coronary angiography or other intervention.

psychosocial: an informal abbreviation used to depict the interplay of psychological (mental) influences and social (including environmental and cultural) influences on human development, behaviour or health.

registrar: the name given to a doctor in training who is given additional responsibilities, usually after completion of pre-vocational training. In hospitals, the position of registrar often involves the oversight and support of interns and other doctors in pre-vocational training.

resident: an abbreviation of resident medical officer. It is an informal term that dates back to a time when junior doctors resided full-time in hospitals. Resident now refers to junior doctors between the intern year and the registrar years (see also junior doctor, pre-vocational training and vocational training).

rotation: see clinical rotation.

senior doctor: a term used in public hospitals to identify a doctor who has completed specialist training, holds the fellowship of the appropriate medical college and is entitled to practise medicine independently and to supervise doctors in training.

vocational training: also known as specialist training; the period spent in postgraduate training to acquire the specific skills and qualifications needed for independent medical practice in a chosen field of medicine.

NOTES

Introduction

1 Available at https://ama.com.au/careers/becoming-a-doctor.

Section 1: Making an informed decision

1 McManus, IC, Livingston, G, Katona, C. 'The attractions of medicine: the generic motivations of medical school applicants in relation to demography, personality and achievement.' *BMC Medical Education*, 2006, 6: 11, www.biomedcentral.com/1472-6920/6/11.

2 *Good Medical Practice: Professionalism, Ethics and Law* (4th edn.). KJ Breen, SM Cordner and CH Thomson. Australian Medical Council, Canberra, 2016.

3 Powis, D. 'Selecting medical students: An unresolved challenge.' *Medical Teacher*, 2015, 37(3): 252–60.

4 Hurwitz, S, Kelly, B, Powis, D et al. 'The desirable qualities of future doctors – a study of medical student perceptions.' *Medical Teacher*, 2013, 35: e1332–9.

5 It is accessible at https://www.medicalboard.gov.au/Codes-Guidelines-Policies/Code-of-conduct.aspx.

6 https://www.medicalboard.gov.au/Codes-Guidelines-Policies/Social-media-policy.aspx.

7 Benbassat, J, Baumal, R. 'Uncertainties in the selection of applicants for medical school.' *Advances in Health Sciences Education*, 2007, 12: 509–21.

8 Munir, V. MABEL: doctors shouldn't work in excess of 50 hours per week, https://insightplus.mja.com.au/2018/6/mabel-doctors-shouldnt-work-in-excess-of-50-hours-per-week/. Managing the risks of fatigue in the medical workforce 2016 AMA Safe Hours Audit. Australian Medical Association 2017, https://ama.com.au/system/tdf/documents/v1%202016%20AMA%20Safe%20Hours%20Audit%20Report.pdf?file=1&type=node&id=46763.

9 Scott, A. ANZ – Melbourne Institute Health Sector Report: Specialists, https://melbourneinstitute.unimelb.edu.au/__data/assets/pdf_file/0016/2800141/ANZ-MI-Health-Sector-Report-Specialists-2018.pdf.

10 Chai Cheng, TC, Scott, A, SH Jeon et al. What factors influence the earnings of GPs and medical specialists in Australia? Evidence from the MABEL Survey, 2010, https://melbourneinstitute.unimelb.edu.au/publications/working-papers/search/result?paper=2156327. Connolly, S, Holdcroft, A. The pay gap for women in medicine and academic medicine, 2006, https://www.

medicalwomensfederation.org.uk/images/Daonload_Pay_Gap_Report.pdf

11 Oliver, D. 'Making less popular medical jobs more attractive.' *BMJ*, 2018, 362: k2936.

12 Scott, A, Joyce, CM. 'The future of medical careers.' *Medical Journal of Australia*, 2014, 201: 82–3.

13 Scott, A. The future of the medical workforce, https: //melbourneinstitute. unimelb.edu.au/__data/assets/pdf_file/0008/3069548/ANZ-MI-Health-Sector-Report-Future.pdf.

14 Salisbury, H. 'Why be a doctor?' *BMJ*, 2019, 365: 12153.

15 Allen, I. *Doctors and their careers. A new generation.* London: Policy Studies Institute; 1994. Goel, S, Angeli, F, Dhirar, N et al. 'What motivates medical students to select medical studies: a systematic literature review.' *BMC Medical Education,* 2018; 18: 16, https: //doi.org/10.1186/s12909-018-1123-4.

16 Powell, A, Boakes, J, Slater, P. 'What motivates medical students: How they see themselves and their profession.' *Medical Education.* 1987, 21: 176–82.

17 McManus, IC, Livingston, G, Katona, C. 'The attractions of medicine: the generic motivations of medical school applicants in relation to demography, personality and achievement.' *BMC Medical Education,* 2006, 6: 11, www. biomedcentral.com/1472-6920/6/11.

18 Crimlisk, H, McManus, IC. 'The effect of personal illness experience on career preference in medical students.' *Medical Education,* 1987, 21: 464–7.

19 Valliant, GE, Sobowale, NC, McArthur, C. 'Some psychological vulnerabilities of physicians.' *N Eng J Med,* 1972, 287: 372–5.

20 Firth-Cozens, J and Harrison, J. *How to survive in medicine personally and professionally.* Wiley-Blackwell, 2010, West Sussex.

21 Ibid.

22 Allen I. *Doctors and their careers. A new generation.* London: Policy Studies Institute, 1994.

23 McManus, IC, Iqbal, S, Chandrarajan, A, Ferguson, E and Leaviss, J. 'Unhappiness and dissatisfaction in doctors cannot be predicted by selectors from medical school application forms: A prospective, longitudinal study.' *BMC Medical Education,* 2005, 5: 38, www.biomedcentral.com/1472-6920/5/38.

24 Markwell, AL, Wainer, Z. The health and well-being of junior doctors: insights from a national survey. *Medical Journal of Australia,* 2009, 191: 441–4. Heredia, DC, Rhodes, CS, English, SE et al. The national Junior Medical Officer Welfare Study: a snapshot of intern life in Australia. *Medical Journal of Australia,* 2009, 191: 445.

25 Joyce, MJ, Schurer, S, Scott, A et al. 'Australian doctors' satisfaction with their work: results from the MABEL longitudinal survey of doctors.' *Medical Journal of Australia,* 2011, 194: 30–3.

26 McManus, IC, Keeling, A, Paice, E. 'Stress, burnout and doctors' attitudes to work are determined by personality and learning style: A twelve-year longitudinal study of UK medical graduates.' *BMC Medicine,* 2004, 2: 29, www. biomedcentral.com/1741-7015/2/29.

27 Tyssen, R, Dolatowski, FC, Rovik, JO et al. 'Personality traits and types predict medical school stress: a six-year longitudinal and nationwide study. *Medical Education*, 2007, 41: 781–7.

Section 2:
The medical schools and the university selection processes

1 Medical Education and Training in Australia National Medical Training Advisory Network, December 2017. Table 2.1 https: //hwd.health.gov.au/webapi/ customer/documents/MET%201st%20edition%202016.pdf.

2 Medical Deans Australia New Zealand. Student Statistics and MSOD National Data Reports, 2018 https: //medicaldeans.org.au/resource/msod-national-data-reports/.

3 https://www.amc.org.au/accreditation-and-recognition/assessment-accreditation-primary-medical-programs/.

4 https://www.amsa.org.au/applying4medguide.

5 Rolfe, IE, Ringland, C, Pearson, SA. 'Graduate entry to medical school? Testing some assumptions.' *Medical Education*, 2004, 38: 778–86.

6 DeWitt, D, Canny, BJ, Nitzberg, M et al. 'Medical student satisfaction, coping and burnout in direct-entry versus graduate-entry programmes.' *Medical Education*, 2016, 50 (6): 637–45.

7 Information is available at https://medicaldeans.org.au/data/medical-schools-outcomes-database-reports/.

8 Garvey, G, Rolfe, IE, Pearson, SA et al. 'Indigenous Australian medical students' perceptions of their medical school training.' *Medical Education*, 2009, 43: 1047–55.

9 Australian Medical Education Study. What makes for success in medical education? Synthesis Report. 2005 https: //trove.nla.gov.au/work/37528130.

10 Hills, J, Rolfe, IE, Pearson, SA et al. 'Do junior doctors feel they are prepared for hospital practice? A study of graduates from traditional and non-traditional medical schools.' *Medical Education*, 1998, 32: 19–24.

11 Bleakley, A, Brennan, N. Does undergraduate curriculum design make a difference to readiness to practice as a junior doctor? *Medical Teacher*, 2011, 33: 459–67.

12 Eley, D, Synnott, R, Baker, P, et al. 'A decade of Australian Rural Clinical School graduates – where are they and why?' *Rural and Remote Health*, 2012, 12: 1937. Clark, TR, Freedman, SB, Croft, AJ et al. 'Medical graduates becoming rural doctors: rural background versus extended rural placement.' *Medical Journal of Australia*, 2013, 199 (11): 779–82. McGirr, J, Seal, A, Barnard, A et al. 'The Australian Rural Clinical School (RCS) program supports rural medical workforce: evidence from a cross-sectional study of 12 RCSs.' *Rural and Remote Health*, 2019, 19: 4971.

13 Eley, D, Baker, P. 'Does recruitment lead to retention? Rural Clinical School training experiences and subsequent intern choices.' *Rural Remote Health*, 2006, 6: 511.

14 https://www.amsa.org.au/applying4medguide.

15 See for example https://www.stjohnvic.com.au/training/first-aid-courses.asp.

16 Storey, M, Mercer, A. 'Selection of medical students: an Australian perspective.' *Int Med Journal*, 2005, 35: 647–9.

17 Wong, CXJ, Nelson, AJ, Roberts-Thomson, RL. 'National approaches for medical school entry.' *Medical Journal of Australia*, 2010, 193: 428.

18 Australian Medical Education Study. What makes for success in medical education? Synthesis Report, https: //trove.nla.gov.au/work/37528130.

19 Benbassat, J. 'Assessments of non-academic attributes in applicants for undergraduate medical education: an overview of advantages and limitations.' *Medical Science Educator*, 2019, https: //doi.org/10.1007/s40670-019-00791-5.

20 Shulruf, B, Bagg, W, Begun, M et al. 'The efficacy of medical student selection tools in Australia and New Zealand.' *Medical Journal of Australia*, 2018, 208: 214–18. Puddey, IB, Mercer, A. 'Predicting academic outcomes in an Australian graduate entry medical programme.' *BMC Medical Education*, 2014, 14: 31.

21 Sladek, RM, Bond, MJ, Frost, LK et al. 'Predicting success in medical school: a longitudinal study of common Australian student selection tools.' *BMC Medical Education*, 2016, 16: 187, https: //doi.org/10.1186/s12909-016-0692-3.

22 Patterson, F, Knight, A, Dowell, J, Nicholson, S, Cousans, F, Cleland, J. 'How effective are selection methods in medical education? A systematic review.' *Medical Education*. 2016, 50: 36–60.

23 McManus, IC, Dewberry, C, Nicholson, S et al. 'The UKCAT-12 study: educational attainment, aptitude test performance, demographic and socio-economic contextual factors as predictors of first year outcome in a cross-sectional collaborative study of 12 UK medical schools.' *BMC Medicine*, 2013, 11: 244.

24 Patterson, F, Zibarras, L, Ashworth, V. 'AMEE Guide. Situational judgement tests in medical education and training: research theory and practice: AMEE Guide No. 100.' *Medical Teacher*, 2016, 38(1): 3–17. Lievens, F. 'Adjusting medical school admission: assessing interpersonal skills using situational judgement tests.' *Medical Education*, 2013, 43: 182–9.

25 Lambe, P, Waters C, Bristow D. 'The UK clinical aptitude test: is if a fair test for selecting medical students?' *Medical Teacher*, 2012, 34: 8, e557–65.

26 Griffin, B, Carless, S, Wilson, I. 'The effect of commercial coaching on selection test performance.' *Medical Teacher*, 2013, 35 (4): 295–300.

27 Aldous, CJ, Leeder, SR, Price, J et al. 'A selection test for Australian graduate-entry medical schools.' *Medical Journal of Australia*, 1997, 166: 247–25.

28 https://isat.acer.edu.au/.

29 Pau, A, Jeevaratnam, K, Chen, YS, et al. 'The Multiple Mini-Interview (MMI) for student selection in health professions training – a systematic review.' *Medical Teacher*, 2013, 35: 1027–41.

30 Razack, S, Faremo, S, Drolet, F et al. 'Multiple mini-interviews versus traditional interviews: stakeholder acceptability comparison.' *Medical Education*, 2009, 43: 993–1000.

31 Dr Ruth Slavek, personal communication.

32 See https://www.uow.edu.au/science-medicine-health/schools-entities/medicine/md/admission-information/domestic-applicants/.

33 https://medicaldeans.org.au/md/2018/07/Inherent-Requirements-FINAL-statement_July-2017.pdf.

34 See https://www.humanservices.gov.au/organisations/health-professionals/services/medicare/medicare-benefits-health-professionals/eligibility-access-medicare-benefits/overseas-trained-doctors-and-foreign-graduates-eligibility-requirements.

35 http://www.medicalboard.gov.au/Registration-Standards.aspx.

36 http://www.ielts.org/default.aspx.

37 Griffin, B, Harding, DW, Wilson, IG and Yeomans, ND. 'Does practice make perfect? The effect of coaching and retesting on selection tests used for admission to an Australian medical school.' *Medical Journal of Australia,* 2008, 189: 270–3.

38 Wilkinson, TM, Wilkinson, TJ. 'Preparation courses for a medical admissions test: effectiveness contrasts with opinion.' *Medical Education,* 2013, 47: 417–24.

39 Goulston, K, Oates, K. 'Admission Policy Review. University of Sydney Faculty of Medicine.' March 2009 http: //catalogue.nla.gov.au/Search/Home?lookfor=978-1-74210-088-3&type=isn&limit%5B%5D=&submit=Find

40 McGaghie, WC, Downing, SM, Kubilius, R. 'What is the impact of commercial test preparation courses on medical examination performance?' *Teaching and Learning in Medicine,* 2004, 16: 202–11.

41 Porter, L. The biggest test: passing the medical, https: //www.smh.com.au/education/the-biggest-test-passing-the-medical-20120312-1uubl.html.

42 Griffin, B, Harding, DW, Wilson, IG and Yeomans, ND. 'Does practice make perfect? The effect of coaching and retesting on selection tests used for admission to an Australian medical school.' *Medical Journal of Australia,* 2008, 189: 270–3.

43 For more detail see https://www.studyassist.gov.au/help-loans/commonwealth-supported-places-csps.

44 https://www.health.gov.au/bmpscheme.

45 For information see https://www.bendigobank.com.au/community/scholarships/.

46 See https://www.humanservices.gov.au/individuals/services/centrelink/relocation-scholarship.

47 https://www.jfpp.com.au.

48 https://www.aida.org.au.

49 See https://www.newcastle.edu.au/joint-medical-program/aboriginal-and-torres-strait-islander-students.

50 For information see https://ama.com.au/advocacy/indigenous-peoples-medical-scholarship.

51 For information see https://www.acn.edu.au/scholarships/indigenous-health-scholarships.

52 https://study.unimelb.edu.au/__data/assets/pdf_file/0032/47876/2018-tuition-fees_International-students_TuitionFeeTables_18_April_2018.pdf.

53 https://www.studyinaustralia.gov.au/english/australian-education/education-costs/education-costs-in-australia and https://www.topuniversities.com/student-info/student-finance/how-much-does-it-cost-study-australia.

54 https://melbourneinstitute.unimelb.edu.au/mabel/results-and-publications/reports-and-working-papers.

55 https://www.sbs.com.au/news/the-feed/here-s-how-the-new-hecs-repayment-thresholds-could-affect-you.

56 https://advancemed.com.au/blog/intern-pay/.

57 https: //www1.health.gov.au/internet/main/publishing.nsf/Content/stronger-rural-health-strategy-the-murray-darling-medical-schools-network.

58 https://www.pqa.net.au.

59 https://takecasper.com.
Section 3: The structure and content of the medical course

1 It is available in full at the AMSA website at http://media.amsa.org.au/internal/official_documents/internal_policies/code_of_ethics_2003.pdf.

2 See https://www.jcu.edu.au/__data/assets/pdf_file/0017/201284/JCU-Medical-Code-of-Conduct-1.pdf.

3 Medical Board of Australia. *Good Medical Practice: A Code of Conduct for Doctors in Australia* https: //www.medicalboard.gov.au/Codes-Guidelines-Policies/Code-of-conduct.aspx.

4 Rogers, WA, Mansfield, PR, Braunack-Mayer, AJ and Jureidini, JN. 'The ethics of pharmaceutical industry relationships with medical students.' *Medical Journal of Australia*, 2004, 180: 411–14.

5 Breen, KJ, Cordner, SM, Thomson, CH. *Good Medical Practice: Professionalism, Ethics and Law.* Australian Medical Council, 2016.

6 Australian Medical Education Study. What makes for success in medical education? Synthesis Report, https: //trove.nla.gov.au/work/37528130.

7 Montgomery, K. *How doctors think. Clinical judgement and the practice of medicine.* Oxford University Press, New York, 2006.

8 Koh, GC. 'Revisiting the "Essentials" of problem-based learning.' *Medical Education*, 2016, 50: 596–9.

9 Chiavaroli, NG, Trumble, SC, McColl, GJ. 'The principles of problem-based learning are more important than the method.' *Medical Journal of Australia*, 2013, 199: 588–90.

10 Taylor, D, Miflin, B. 'Problem-based learning: where are we now?' *Medical Teacher*, 2008, 30: 742–63.

11 Koh, GCH, Khoo, HE, Wong, ML et al. 'The effects of problem-based learning during medical school on physician competency: a systematic review.' *Canadian Medical Association Journal*, 208, 178: 3441.

12 Lewis, AD, Menezes, DA, McDermott, HE et al. 'A comparison of stressors in undergraduate problem-based learning (PBL) versus non-PBL medical programmes.' *BMC Medical Education*, 2009; Sep. 13, 9: 60.

13　Australian Medical Education Study. What makes for success in medical education? Synthesis Report, https: //trove.nla.gov.au/work/37528130.

14　Chiavaroli, NG, Trumble, SC, McColl, GJ. 'The principles of problem-based learning are more important than the method.' *Medical Journal of Australia,* 2013, 199: 588–90.

15　https://ama.com.au/position-statement/code-ethics-2004-editorially-revised-2006-revised-2016.

16　Waterman, LZ, Weinman, JA. 'Medical student syndrome: fact or fiction? A cross-sectional study.' *JRSM Open,* 2014 Feb., 5(2): doi: 10.1177/2042533313512480.

17　Scott, KM, Caldwell, PHY, Barnes, EH et al. '"Teaching by humiliation" and mistreatment of medical students in clinical rotations: a pilot study.' *Medical Journal of Australia,* 2015, 203 (4): 185e 1–6.

18　Vogel, L. 'Bullying still rife in medical training.' *Canadian Medical Association Journal,* 2016, 188 (5): 321–2.

19　Timm, A. '"It would not be tolerated in any other profession except medicine": survey reporting on undergraduates' exposure to bullying and harassment in their first placement year.' *BMJ Open,* 2014, 4(7): e005140.

20　Hafferty, FW. 'Beyond curriculum reform: confronting medicine's hidden curriculum.' *Academic Medicine,* 1998, 73: 403–7. Martimianakis, A, Michalec, B, Lam, J, et al. 'Humanism, the hidden curriculum, and educational reform: A scoping review and thematic analysis.' *Academic Medicine,* 2015, 90 (11 Suppl): S5–S13.

21　Hicks, LK, Lin, Y, Robertson, DL and Woodrow, SI. 'Understanding the ethical dilemmas that shape medical students' ethical development: questionnaire survey and focus group study.' *BMJ,* 2001, 322: 709–10.

22　Kushner, TK, Thomasma, DC (eds). *Ward Ethics: Dilemmas for Medical Students and Doctors in Training.* Cambridge University Press, Cambridge, 2001.

23　Braunack-Mayer AJ. 'Should medical students act as surrogate patients for each other?' *Medical Education,* 2001, 35: 681–6. Outram, S, Nair, BR. 'Peer physical examination: time to revisit?' *Medical Journal of Australia,* 2008, 189: 274–6.

24　Koehler, N., McMenamin, C. 'The need for a peer physical examination policy within Australian medical schools.' *Medical Teacher,* 2014, 36 (5): 430–3.

25　Bai, M, Nicholson, H, Smith-Han, K. 'Medical students' experiences of practising medical procedures on patients, other students and themselves.' *NZ Med J,* 2016, 129(1444): 43–57.

26　Gerber, LA. *Married to their careers.* Tavistock Publications, New York, 1983.

27　Medical Deans Australia New Zealand. *Inherent requirements for studying medicine in Australia and New Zealand,* https: //documents.uow.edu.au/content/groups/public/@web/@smah/@med/documents/doc/uow219416.pdf.

28　Elton, C. *Also human: The inner lives of doctors,* 2018, Penguin Random House, UK.

29　More detailed information is available at https://www.ahpra.gov.au/Registration/Student-Registrations.aspx.

30 Papadakis, MA, Teherani, A, Banach, MA et al. 'Disciplinary action by medical boards and prior behaviour in medical school.' *NEJM*, 2005, 353: 2673–82.

31 Mak-van der Vossen, M, van Mook, W, van der Burgt, S, et al. 'Descriptors for unprofessional behaviours of medical students: a systematic review and categorisation.' *BMC Medical Education*, 2017, 17: 164.

32 McGurgan, PM, Olson-White, D, Holgate, M and Carmody, D. 'Fitness-to-practise policies in Australian medical schools – are they fit for purpose?' *Medical Journal of Australia*, 2010, 193: 665–7.

33 Parker, MH, Turner, J, McGurgan, P et al. 'The difficult problem: assessing medical students' professional attitudes and behaviour.' *Medical Journal of Australia*, 2010, 193: 662–4.

Section 4: The reality of life as a medical student

1   Australian Medical Education Study. What makes for success in medical education? Synthesis Report, https: //trove.nla.gov.au/work/37528130.

2   Ibid.

3   Firth, J. 'Levels and sources of stress in medical students.' *BMJ*, 1986, 292, 1177–80. Ishak W, Nikravesh, R, Lederer, S, et al. 'Burnout in medical students: a systematic review.' *Clinical Teacher*, 2013, 10(4): 242–5. Dyrbye, L, Shanafelt, T. 'A narrative review on burnout experienced by medical students and residents.' *Medical Education*, 2016 Jan., 50(1): 132–49.

4   White, GE. 'Sexual harassment during medical training: the perception of medical students at a university medical school on Australia.' *Medical Education*, 2000, 34: 980–6.

5   Wilkinson, TJ, Gill, DJ, Fitzjohn, J, et al. 'The impact on students of adverse experiences during medical education.' *Medical Teacher*, 2006, 28: 101–2.

6   Jones, GI, DeWitt, DE, Cross, M. 'Medical students' perceptions of barriers to training at a rural clinical school.' *Rural Remote Health*, 2007, 7: 685.

7   Firth-Cozens, J. 'Medical student stress.' *Medical Education*, 2001, 35: 6–7.

8   Tyssen, R, Dolanski, FC, Rovik, JO et al. 'Personality traits and types predict medical school stress: a six-year longitudinal and nationwide study.' *Medical Education*, 2007, 41: 781–7.

9   Doherty, EM, Nugent, E. 'Personality factors and medical training: a review of the literature.' *Medical Education*, 2011, 45: 132–40.

10 Firth-Cozens, J. Harrison, J. *How to survive in medicine, personally and professionally*. Oxford, Wiley-Blackwell, 2010.

11 Willcock, SM, Daly, MG, Tennant, CC and Allard, BJ. 'Burnout and psychiatric morbidity in new medical graduates.' *Medical Journal of Australia*, 2004, 181: 357–60.

12 DeWitt, D, Canny, BJ, Nitzberg, M et al. 'Medical student satisfaction, coping and burnout in direct-entry versus graduate-entry programmes.' *Medical Education*, 2016, 50 (6): 637–45.

13 Casey, D, Thomas, S, Hocking, DR et al. 'Graduate-entry medical students: older

and wiser but not less distressed.' *Australasian Psychiatry*, 2016, 24(1): 88–92.

14 Wagner, RE, Hexel, M, Bauer, WW and Kropiunigg, U. 'Crying in hospitals: A survey of doctors', nurses' and medical students' experiences and attitudes.' *Medical Journal of Australia*, 1997, 166: 13–6.

15 Sung, AD, Collins, ME, Smith, AK et al. 'Crying: experiences and attitudes of third-year medical students and interns.' *Teaching and Learning in Medicine*, 2009, 21: 180–7.

16 Benbassat, J, Baumal, R, Chan, S and Nirel, N. 'Sources of distress during medical training and clinical practice: Suggestions for reducing their impact.' *Medical Teacher*, 2011, 33(6): 486–90.

17 Benbassat J. 'Undesirable features of the medical learning environment: a narrative review of the literature.' *Advances in Health Sciences Education. Theory and Practice*, 2013, 18(3): 527–36.

18 https://www.amsa.org.au/node/948.

19 Brazeau, CM, Schroeder, R, Rovi, S et al. 'Relationships between medical student burnout, empathy, and professionalism climate.' *Academic Medicine*, 2010, 85 (10 Suppl): S33–6.

20 Dyrbye, L, Shanafelt, T. 'A narrative review on burnout experienced by medical students and residents.' *Medical Education*, 2016 Jan., 50(1): 132–49.

21 Dyrbye, LN, Massie, FS, Eacker, A et al. 'Relationship between burnout and professional conduct and attitudes among US medical students.' *JAMA*, 2010, 304: 1173–80.

22 Santen, SA, Holt, DB, Kemp, JD and Hemphill, RR. 'Burnout in medical students: examining the prevalence and associated factors.' *Southern Medical Journal*, 2010, 103: 758–63. Dahlin, M, Fjell, J, Runeson, B. 'Factors at medical school and work related to exhaustion among physicians in their first postgraduate year.' *Nordic Journal of Psychiatry*, 2010, 64 (6): 402–8.

23 Hassed, C, de Lisle, S, Sullivan, G and Pier, C. 'Enhancing the health of medical students: outcomes of an integrated mindfulness and lifestyle program.' *Advances in Health Sciences Education*, 2008, 14: 387–98.

24 Kjeldstadii, K, Tyssen, R, Finset, F et al. 'Life satisfaction and resilience in medical school – a six year longitudinal, nationwide and comparative study.' *BMC Medical Education*, 2006 Sep., 19, 6: 48.

25 Australian Medical Students' Association. *Keeping Your Grass Greener: A Wellbeing Guide for Medical Students*, http: //mentalhealth.amsa.org.au/wp-content/uploads/2014/08/KYGGWebVersion.pdf.

26 Tyssen, R, Vaglum, P, Grenvold, NT and Ekeberg, O. 'Factors in medical school that predict postgraduate mental health problems in need of treatment. A nationwide and longitudinal study.' *Medical Education*, 2001, 35: 110–20.

27 https://www.beyondblue.org.au/docs/default-source/research-project-files/bl1132-report---nmhdmss-full-report_web.

28 Matheson, KM, Barrett, T, Landine, J et al. 'Experiences of psychological distress and sources of stress and support during medical training: a survey of medical students.' *Academic Psychiatry*, 2016: 40 (1), 63–8.

29 Tam, W, Lo K Pacheco, J. 'Prevalence of depressive symptoms among medical students: overview of systematic reviews.' *Medical Education,* 2019, 53 (4): 345–54.

30 Schwenk, TL, Davis, L, Wimsatt, LA. 'Depression, stigma and suicidal ideation in medical students.' *JAMA,* 2010, 304: 1181–90. Roberts, LW. 'Understanding depression and distress among medical students.' *JAMA,* 2010, 304: 1231–3.

31 Hillis, JM, Perry, WR, Carroll, EY et al. 'Painting the picture: Australasian medical student views on wellbeing teaching and support services.' *Medical Journal of Australia,* 2010, 192: 188–90.

32 http://www.vdhp.org.au/website/home.html.

33 http://dhas.org.au/.

34 http://dhas.org.au/contact/contact-dhas-in-other-states-territories-and-new-zealand.html.

35 Australian Medical Students' Association. *Keeping Your Grass Greener: A Wellbeing Guide for Medical Students,* http: //mentalhealth.amsa.org.au/wp-content/uploads/2014/08/KYGGWebVersion.pdf

36 https://medicaldeans.org.au/md/2001/07/Infectious-Disease-Policy.pdf.

37 Communicable Diseases Network Australia. *Australian National Guidelines for the Management of Healthcare Workers Living with Blood Borne Viruses and Healthcare Workers who Perform Exposure Prone Procedures at Risk of Exposure to Blood Borne Viruses,* https: //www1.health.gov.au/internet/main/publishing.nsf/Content/cda-cdna-bloodborne.htm.

38 Mitchell, BG, Shaban, RZ, MacBeth, D et al. 'The burden of healthcare-associated infection in Australian hospitals: A systematic review of the literature.' *Infection, Disease & Health,* 2017, 22: 117–28.

39 Sladek, RM, Bond, MJ, Phillips, PA. 'Why don't doctors wash their hands? A correlational study of thinking styles and hand hygiene.' *American Journal of Infection Control,* 2008, 36 (6): 399–406.

40 Evans, D, Brown, J. *How to succeed at medical school. An essential guide to learning.* Wiley-Blackwell BMJ Books, UK, 2009.

41 http://mentalhealth.amsa.org.au/wp-content/uploads/2014/08/KYGGWebVersion.pdf.

Section 5:
The intern year and beyond: Career paths for medical graduates

1 A successful intern job share. AMA Victoria, https: //amavic.com.au/stethoscope/-95-a-successful-intern-job-share.

2 See https://advancemed.com.au/blog/intern-pay/.

3 Australian Medical Education Study. What makes for success in medical education? Synthesis Report, 2005, https: //trove.nla.gov.au/work/37528130.

4 Joint AMC–MBA Preparedness for Internship Survey 2018, https: //www.amc.org.au/accreditation-and-recognition/assessment-accreditation-primary-medical-programs/joint-amc-mba-preparedness-for-internship-survey/.

5 https://www.medicaltrainingsurvey.gov.au/.

6   Review of medical intern training 2015. Commissioned by the Australian Health Ministers' Advisory Council, www.coaghealthcouncil.gov.au/medicalinternreview.

7   https://www.amsa.org.au/amsa-internship-guide-2019.

8   https://ama.com.au/resources/doctors-in-training.

9   https://www.amc.org.au/accreditation-and-recognition/assessment-accreditation-prevocational-phase-medical-education/national-internship-framework/.

10 https://www.medicalboard.gov.au/Registration/Interns/Guidelines-resources-tools.aspx.

11 https://www.amsa.org.au/amsa-internship-guide-2019.

12 Report on the National Audit of Applications and Acceptances for Medical Internship and the Late Vacancy Management Process for 2017 Clinical Year, http://www.coaghealthcouncil.gov.au/Portals/0/Report%20on%20the%20National%20Audit%20of%20Applications%20and%20Acceptances%20for%20Medical%20Internship%20and%20the%20Late%20Vacancy%20Management%20Process%20for%202017%20Clinical%20Year.pdf.

13 See http://www.cpmec.org.au for links to all these websites.

14 Ryan, AT, Ewing, HP, O'Brien, RC. 'Practice interviews for final-year medical students.' *Medical Education,* 2014, 48 (5): 528–9.

15 Heredia, DC, Rhodes, CS, English, SE et al. 'The national Junior Medical Officer Welfare Study: a snapshot of intern life in Australia.' *Medical Journal of Australia,* 2009, 191: 445.

16 Markwell, AL, Wainer, Z. 'The health and well-being of junior doctors: insights from a national survey.' *Medical Journal of Australia,* 2009, 191: 441–4.

17 Willcock, SM, Daly, MG, Tennant, CC and Allard, BJ. 'Burnout and psychiatric morbidity in new medical graduates.' *Medical Journal of Australia,* 2004, 181: 357–60.

18 Dyrbye, L, Shanafelt, T. 'A narrative review on burnout experienced by medical students and residents.' *Medical Education,* 2016 Jan., 50(1): 132–49.

19 Brennan, N, Corrigan, O, Allard, J et al. 'The transition from medical student to junior doctor: today's experiences of tomorrow's doctors.' *Medical Education,* 2010, 44: 449–58. Firth-Cozens, J, Harrison, J. *How to survive in medicine personally and professionally.* Wiley-Blackwell, 2010, West Sussex.

20 Westbrook, J, Sunderland, N, Victoria Atkinson, V et al. 'Endemic unprofessional behaviour in health care: the mandate for a change in approach.' *Medical Journal of Australia,* 2018, 209 (9): 380–2. Westbrook, J, Sunderland, N. Bullying and harassment of health workers endangers patient safety, https://theconversation.com/bullying-and-harassment-of-health-workers-endangers-patient-safety-106167. Rowe, L. Endemic bullying: narcissistic personality disorder in medicine, https://insightplus.mja.com.au/2019/9/endemic-bullying-narcissistic-personality-disorder-in-medicine/. Coopes, A. 'Operate with respect: how Australia is confronting sexual harassment of trainees.' *BMJ,* 2018, 354: i4210. Llewellyn, A, Karageorge, B, Nash et al. 'Bullying and sexual harassment of junior doctors in New South Wales, Australia: rate and reporting outcomes.' *Australian Health Review,* 2018, 43(3): 328–34.

21 Levi, E. The dark side of doctoring, http: //medicalrepublic.com.au/dark-side-doctoring/9065.

22 Firth-Cozens, J, Harrison J. *How to survive in medicine personally and professionally.* Wiley-Blackwell, 2010, West Sussex.

23 Tyssen, R, Vaglum, P, Grenvold, NT et al. 'The relative importance of individual and organisational factors for the prevention of job stress during internship: a nationwide and prospective study.' *Medical Teacher,* 2005, 27: 726–31.

24 Dahlin, M, Fjell, J and Runeson, B. 'Factors at medical school and work related to exhaustion among physicians in their first postgraduate year.' *Nordic Journal of Psychiatry,* 2010, 64: 402–8.

25 Launer, J. 'Resilience: for and against.' *Postgraduate Medical Journal,* 2015, 91: 721–2. Peters, D, Horn, C, Gishen, F. 'Ensuring our future doctors are resilient.' *BMJ,* 2018, 362: k2877.

26 Vogel, L. 'Even resilient doctors report high levels of burnout, finds CMA survey.' *Canadian Medical Association Journal,* 2018, 190 (43): E1293. Huntington GR. 'Resilience training is a slap in the face.' *BMJ,* 2019, 365: l4176. Balme, E, Gerada, C, Page, L. 'Doctors need to be supported, not trained in resilience.' *BMJ Careers,* 15 Sep. 2015, http: //careers.bmj.com.ezproxy.lib.monash.edu.au/careers/advice/Doctors_need_to_be_supported,_not_trained_in_resilience. Thiemt, D. 'Resilience training is just a band-aid solution for doctor well-being: Yes.' *Emergency Medicine Australasia,* 2018, 30(2): 259–60.

27 Forbes, M, Byrom, L, van der Steenstraten, I et al. 'Resilience on the run – an evaluation of a wellbeing program for medical interns.' *Internal Medicine Journal,* 2019, Apr. 16, doi: 10.1111/imj.14324.

28 Dyrbye, LN, Satele, D, Shanafelt, TD. 'Healthy exercise habits are associated with lower risk of burnout and higher quality of life among U.S. medical students.' *Academic Medicine,* 2017, 92 (7): 1006–11.

29 Paice, E, Hamilton-Fairley, D. 'Avoiding burnout in new doctors: sleep, supervision and teams.' *Postgraduate Medical Journal,* 2013, 89: 493–4.

30 Spinelli, C, Wisener, M, Khoury, B. 'Mindfulness training for healthcare professionals and trainees: A meta-analysis of randomized controlled trials.' *Journal of Psychosomatic Research,* 2019, 120: 29–38.

31 Mahmood, J, Grotmol, K, Tesli, M et al. 'Risk factors measured during medical school for later hazardous drinking: A 10-year, longitudinal, nationwide study.' *Alcohol and Alcoholism,* 2016, 51 (1): 71–6.

32 Chanchlani, S, Chang, D, Ong, J et al. 'The value of peer mentoring for the psychosocial wellbeing of junior doctors: a randomised controlled study.' *Medical Journal of Australia,* 2018, 209 (9): 401–5.

33 Firth-Cozens, J, Harrison, J. *How to survive in medicine personally and professionally.* Wiley-Blackwell, 2010, West Sussex. Gerber, LA. *Married to their careers.* Tavistock Publications, New York, 1983.

34 https://ama.com.au/article/national-code-practice-hours-work-shiftwork-and-rostering-hospital-doctors.

35 https://ama.com.au/article/2016-ama-safe-hours-audit.

36 Robson, S. 'Learn from me.' *MJA Insight,* https: //insightplus.mja.com. au/2018/41/learn-from-me-speak-out-seek-help-get-treatment/.

37 Elton, C. *Also human: The inner lives of doctors,* 2018, Penguin Random House, UK.

38 Foster, K, Roberts, C. 'The heroic and the villainous: a qualitative study characterising the role models that shaped senior doctors' professional identity.' *BMC Medical Education,* 2016, 16 (1): 206. Benbassat, J. 'Role modelling in medical education: The importance of reflective imitation.' *Academic Medicine,* 2014, 89: 550–4.

39 McCartney, M. 'Reading makes us better doctors.' *BMJ,* 2018, 362: k3373.

40 Dyrbye, LN, Satele, D, Shanafelt, TD. 'Healthy exercise habits are associated with lower risk of burnout and higher quality of life among U.S. medical students.' *Academic Medicine,* 2017, 92 (7): 1006–11.

41 Paice, E, Hamilton-Fairley, D. 'Avoiding burnout in new doctors: sleep, supervision and teams.' *Postgraduate Medical Journal,* 2013, 89: 493–4.

42 Markwell, AL, Wainer, Z. 'The health and well-being of junior doctors: insights from a national survey.' *Medical Journal of Australia,* 2009, 191: 441–4. Heredia, DC, Rhodes, CS, English, SE et al. 'The national Junior Medical Officer Welfare Study: a snapshot of intern life in Australia.' *Medical Journal of Australia,* 2009, 191: 445.

43 Dr Ashley Watson, personal communication.

44 Cooke, L, Chitty, A. Why do doctors leave the profession? British Medical Association. Health Policy and Economic Research Unit 2004 – quoted by Elton, p. 350.

45 Elton, C. *Also human: The inner lives of doctors.* 2018, Penguin Random House, UK.

46 Veitch, C, Underhill A, Hays RB. 'The career aspirations and location intentions of James Cook University's first cohort of medical students: a longitudinal study at course entry and graduation.' *Rural Remote Health,* 2006, 6(1): 537.

47 See https://ama.com.au/careers/becoming-a-doctor.

48 www.agpt.com.au.

49 Egan, JM, Webber, MGT, King, MRD et al. 'The hospitalist: a third alternative.' *Medical Journal of Australia,* 2000, 172: 335–8.

50 Hillman, K. 'The hospitalist: a US model ripe for importing?' *Medical Journal of Australia,* 2003, 178: 54–5.

51 Australian Medical Education Study. What makes for success in medical education? Synthesis Report, 2005, https: //trove.nla.gov.au/work/37528130.

52 https://www.mapmycareer.health.nsw.gov.au/Pages/explore.aspx?section=ms.

53 See https://www.racgp.org.au/become-a-gp/general-practice-career-guide.

54 Stagg, P, Prideaux, D, Greenhill, J, Sweet, L. 'Are medical students influenced by preceptors in making career choices, and if so how? A systematic review.' *Rural Remote Health,* 2012, 12: 1832.

55 Grigg, M, Arora, M, Diwan AD. 'Australian medical students and their choice of

surgery as a career: a review.' *ANZ Journal of Surgery*, 2014, 84: 653–5.

56 Heikkilä, T, Hyppölä, H, Kumpusalo, E et al. 'Choosing a medical specialty – Study of Finnish doctors graduating in 1977–2006.' *Medical Teacher*, 2011, 33: e440–5.

57 Smith, F, Lambert, TW, Goldacre, MJ. 'Factors influencing junior doctors' choices of future specialty: trends over time and demographics based on results from UK national surveys.' *Journal of the Royal Society of Medicine*, 2015, 108: 396–405.

58 Sivey, P, Scott, A, Witt, J et al. 'Junior doctors' preferences for specialty choice.' *Journal of Health Economics*, 2012, 31: 813–23.

59 Elton, C. *Also human: The inner lives of doctors*. 2018, Penguin Random House, UK.

60 Harris, MG, Gavel, PH, Young, JR. 'Factors influencing the choice of specialty of Australian medical graduates.' *Medical Journal of Australia*, 2005, 183: 295–300.

61 Kassamali, R, Gill, C, Murphy, A, et al. 'Finding direction: What influences medical students in their final career speciality choices?' *Medical Teacher*, 2013, 35: 339.

62 Harris, MG, Gavel, PH and Young, JR. 'Factors influencing the choice of specialty of Australian medical graduates.' *Medical Journal of Australia*, 2005, 183: 295–300.

63 Firth-Cozens, J, Harrison, J. *How to survive in medicine personally and professionally*. Wiley-Blackwell, 2010, West Sussex.

64 Considine, NS, Yu, TC, Hill, AG et al. 'Disgust sensitivity and the 'non-rational' aspects of a career choice in surgery.' *New Zealand Medical Journal*, 2013, 126: 19–26.

65 See https://melbourneinstitute.unimelb.edu.au/mabel/results-and-publications.

66 Sivey, P, Scott, A, Witt, J, Joyce, C and Humphreys, J. 2010. Why junior doctors don't want to become general practitioners: A discrete choice experiment from the MABEL longitudinal study of doctors. Melbourne Institute Working Paper No. 17/10.

67 Scott, A. The future of the medical workforce, https: //melbourneinstitute. unimelb.edu.au/__data/assets/pdf_file/0008/3069548/ANZ-MI-Health-Sector-Report-Future.pdf.

68 Tolhurst, HM, Stewart, SM. 'Balancing work, family and other lifestyle aspects: a qualitative study of Australian medical students' attitudes.' *Medical Journal of Australia*, 2004, 181: 361–4.

69 Lennon, M, O'Sullivan, B, McGrail, M et al. 'Attracting junior doctors to rural centres: A national study of work-life conditions and satisfaction.' *Australian Journal of Rural Health*, https: //onlinelibrary.wiley.com/doi/full/10.1111/ ajr.12577.

70 Elton, C. *Also human: The inner lives of doctors*. 2018, Penguin Random House, UK.

71 Scott, A. The future of the medical workforce, https: //melbourneinstitute. unimelb.edu.au/__data/assets/pdf_file/0008/3069548/ANZ-MI-Health-Sector-Report-Future.pdf.

72 See for example https://www.aihw.gov.au/reports-data/health-welfare-services/ workforce/overview.

73 Roberts, C, Togno, JM. 'Selection into specialist training programs: an approach from general practice.' *Medical Journal of Australia,* 2011, 194: 93–5.

74 Duckett, SJ and Willcox, S. *The Australian Health Care System.* 5th edn. Oxford University Press, Melbourne, 2015.

INDEX

Printed in Australia
Ingram Content Group Australia Pty Ltd
AUHW020046251124
403249AU00003B/71